Praise for *You Were*

As a general surgeon with more than thirty years of experience in healthcare, I truly believe that this book is a "must-read." The prevalence of Alzheimer's disease is such that we will all interact with it at some point in our families or chosen professions. Marianne does a remarkable job of intertwining her personal experiences with her grandmother and mother—and the medical and scientific facts and data about Alzheimer's disease—in a way that demonstrates the challenges faced by loved ones and caregivers alike. As I read and noted how Benz and her family approached the disease in "Ma" (her grandmother), and her mother completely differently, it reinforced an axiom I have used in caring for my patients over the past three decades—the need to "meet people where they are." In her case, it truly enabled Benz to describe how her understanding of the challenges allowed her to embrace the love and admiration she had for her mother as she progressed through the stages of the disease. A lesson for all of us...

— Eric S. Bour, MD, MBA, FACS

You Were Still Dancing is an honest guide for navigating the rollercoaster ride that is Alzheimer's. Marianne Benz straps the reader in for the many ups and downs and terrifying loops this tragic condition presents to everyone involved. Benz mixes humor, truth, sadness, and pain as she empties her soul onto the pages of her book and leads her readers down a path of hope with the fighting spirit of a loving daughter who won't accept NO for her precious mother. Her raw honesty will elicit visceral reactions from readers and allow them to peel away each layer of grief as she details not only her struggles but a tragic history of struggles. As a registered nurse with a history in neuroscience, I praise the level of scientific detail Benz includes about this complex condition. This is a textbook on how to navigate the challenges and horrors of an Alzheimer's demise. I recommend this book to anyone who seeks acceptance and validation that it is OK to feel a storm of conflicting emotions when caring for a loved one with Alzheimer's.

— Sally Bartlett, RN, BSN

For years I have experienced Marianne's gift of hospitality. She creates welcoming spaces where others feel seen, wanted, and cared for. She does this in her home. She does this on the go. And now with her book, she's done it through her life, inviting us into her intimate journey with Alzheimer's. It's a generous welcome, and as usual, she makes it accessible and real. On any unknown path with difficult terrain, I look for wise guides. Through this story, Marianne reveals herself as such. She enters courageously with her whole self—mind, heart, body, and world of relationships. Her desire for more, for her mom and herself, is a light that leads her, and us, if we choose to listen, towards exactly that in surprising ways. Marianne shows us what it looks likes on ground level to choose courage and compassion on a journey, while not denying real pain, fear, and loss. Her story gives evidence to the reality that life can come from death, whether that be a literal death or something that feels like a death sentence. And that sometimes this new life emerges by holding on and perhaps more often, by letting go. I leave these pages feeling hopeful and moved by a tenacious love that transforms both those we seek to love well, and ourselves in the process.

— Juli Able, Spiritual Director and author of *A Brilliant Night: Experiencing God in the Hard, Unexpected, and Unfinished*

Despite a heart bursting with mother-daughter love, and a sorely tested spirit, Benz leads her readers forward with the strength and tenacity of a seasoned prima ballerina. Somehow, still light-footed and encouraging, the author acts as both guide and explorer, sharing ups and downs as she narrates a poetic waltz no child *wants* to imagine, let alone take part in. *You Were Still Dancing* presents a thoughtfully woven braid of scientific reasoning, spiritual sensitivity, and emotional intelligence, as the author details her own deeply personal saga with her mother's Alzheimer's in a straightforward, boots on the ground kind of way. Benz leaves no omen or obstacle, no obligation or observance, and no emotion—from joy to devastation—untouched. An impossibly tough topic handled with stunning clarity and extraordinary grace.

— Deborah Mantella, author of *My Sweet Vidalia*

You Were Still Dancing

AN UNFORGETTABLE JOURNEY THROUGH ALZHEIMER'S

Marianne Benz

Christmas Lake Press

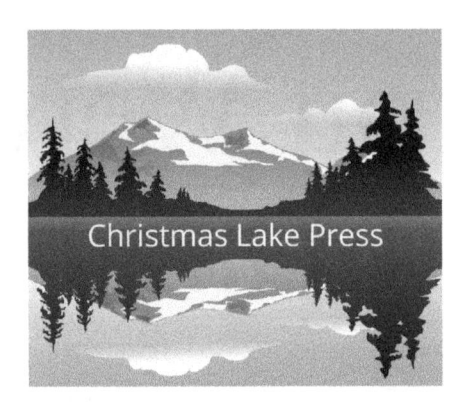

Published by Christmas Lake Press 2024
www.christmaslakecreative.com

Copyright © 2024 by Marianne Benz

ISBN 978-1-960865-20-5

All rights reserved. No part of this publication may be reproduced, stored in a retrieval system, or transmitted in any form, or by any means, electronic, mechanical, photocopying, recording, or otherwise without the prior permission in writing of the copyright holder, nor be otherwise circulated in any form or binding or cover other than in which it is published without a similar condition being imposed on the subsequent publisher.

Interior layout by Daiana Marchesi

You Were Still Dancing

Dedication

To Mom and Ma

Acknowledgments

First, I would like to thank my husband, and best friend of over forty years, Steve, without whose encouragement, support, and love, my story might only exist within the files of my One Drive, and my free time would still be spent editing, researching, more editing, more... I'd become very content in the process of hunkering down in front of my computer, wrapped in a cozy throw, writing, searching the latest articles on Alzheimer's, and drinking lattes. But you pushed me out of my comfort zone, and beyond a pastime to find a publisher and finally set this message free. You are the true wings beneath this publication!

Ryan, Brady, and Drew—there was never a dull moment after you entered our world, but nor was there more joy or meaning in life. Thank you for your generous gift of love to Memaw over the course of your lives with her, but especially after she became sick and seemed to forget who you were. You never treated her any differently after she was sick, and I am certain your love continued to break through the barriers Alzheimer's erected in her. Jody, Christienne, and Darian, thank you from the bottom of my heart for loving my sons and grandkids so well! I probably bored all of you to tears over the years with my chatter about Mom and Ma, but thanks for listening, for your inspirations, for critiquing chapters, and to you Drew for professional advice on all things medical, especially reputable research links.

To my siblings, their spouses, and families, who continued to show up long after Mom had forgotten your names. All of you were instrumental in not only seeing her through the tough times in Cincy, but your physical presence and phone calls after she moved to Atlanta supported her, and me, in ways too numerous to mention… especially you, Cathy Biggs. Mom and Dad would be so proud of the loving, extended family they created and that continues to grow!

To Deborah Mantella (a fellow author who assisted us on the final readthrough), and Jean Ryckman, for your love and support over the decades—with Mom, this book, and all things life. Although our moms are gone, the memories of lunch dates with them in their twilight years that were so fun, *and* funny, will live on in our hearts!

To Denise Vaughn, whose loyal and loving friendship has remained—through the miles—since our camp counselor days. When I count my numerous blessings, you're DOUBLE :)

To my friend Janice St. Hilaire who has echoed so many of my life circumstances—and I hers. Thank you for your ongoing inspiration of a grace filled life, especially when life brings challenges.

To my Thursday morning Bible study ladies, who walked my journey with Mom, lockstep with me, as you supported and prayed for me. And to Juli Able, spiritual director, author, and leader of our study—you continue to be a source of spiritual inspiration to me.

To all those who lovingly cared for Mom, in my home, and in assisted living and memory care. Your work is a calling to minister to those in the trenches, and I especially thank you for loving my mom through all of the unpleasantness of Alzheimer's.

To the Alzheimer's and dementia support groups I attended that provided me with the information and courage I so desperately needed for the road ahead.

To my sister-in-law, Dawn Benz, a fellow partner in crime and author who's knocking out children's books faster than I can write this. You inspire me to continue writing!

To Ericka McIntyre, my first developmental editor. Thank you for your expertise on the developmental and technical aspects of writing that began the process of fitting the pieces of this puzzle together.

To my beta readers, Eric Bour, MD, MBA, FACS; Deborah Mantella; Sally Bartlett, RN; and Juli Able; thank you for your generosity in reading and reviewing this manuscript.

And last, but certainly not least, to the incredibly professional and talented team at Christmas Lake Press: Publisher (and developmental editor) Thomas Fiffer, Copyeditor Parker Gordon, typesetter Daiana Marchesi, and cover designer Katarina Naskovsky, who helped me turn this manuscript into a living, breathing verb— a message of light that continues to shine against the backdrop of darkness which we know as Alzheimer's. Thomas, I will miss our months and months of developmental editing, and our Thursday morning Zoom calls and discussions, but mostly, I will always be grateful for your gentle prodding for me to go deeper, to expand on my thoughts and words, and to help me bring out the very best version of this book.

Alone we can do so little, together we can do so much.
— Helen Keller

Contents

Preface..xix

Prologue..xxi

Chapter One
    Where It All Began..1

Chapter Two
    This Thing Called Memory.......................................7

Chapter Three
    A Bit about Ma..15

Chapter Four
    She's Running Away..19

Chapter Five
    The Entertaining Moments of Alzheimer's.......................29

Chapter Six
    A (Not So) Novel Disease......................................39

CHAPTER SEVEN
The Nightmare Begins..43

CHAPTER EIGHT
The Final Goodbye..49

CHAPTER NINE
The Beginning of the Bizarre..57

CHAPTER TEN
What I Wish I Knew Then (The Latest Data on Alzheimer's)...67

CHAPTER ELEVEN
The Bizarre Has a Name...75

CHAPTER TWELVE
The Game Changer..83

CHAPTER THIRTEEN
The Conversation and the Fall......................................89

CHAPTER FOURTEEN
Home Redefined..97

CHAPTER FIFTEEN
Could It Be This Easy?..107

CHAPTER SIXTEEN
The Hostage Situation...115

CHAPTER SEVENTEEN
The Bad Guy..123

CHAPTER EIGHTEEN
Call in the Troops..147

CHAPTER NINETEEN
The Tough Decision..153

CHAPTER TWENTY
It's All Coming Together...163

CHAPTER TWENTY-ONE
A New Life Is Born...169

CHAPTER TWENTY-TWO
Learning to Be Carried..173

CHAPTER TWENTY-THREE
Apprehended by Awe..179

CHAPTER TWENTY-FOUR
Saved by Friendship..183

CHAPTER TWENTY-FIVE
Patty Re-Invented..193

CHAPTER TWENTY-SIX
Fighting the Establishment......................................197

CHAPTER TWENTY-SEVEN
Moving Upstairs..205

CHAPTER TWENTY-EIGHT
A Word about Fear..213

Chapter Twenty-Nine
From the Physical to the Spiritual..................219

Chapter Thirty
If It Gets Too Tough, Mom, It's OK to Let Go................225

Chapter Thirty-One
No Room at the Inn.......................239

Chapter Thirty-Two
The Gang's All Here......................247

Chapter Thirty-Three
Moving Day, Monday......................251

Chapter Thirty-Four
A Brief Visit, Sunday......................259

Chapter Thirty-Five
Shortly after Sunset......................273

Epilogue..................277

Endnotes..................283

Preface

If you change the way you look at things, the things you look at change.
WAYNE DYER

When Alzheimer's seized my mom, decades after her own mother died of the same disease, differing beliefs—even within myself—came into play over whether or not Mom still existed within her failing cognition. Our ensuing and surprising journey, I believe, was largely influenced by an openness to see beyond my mind's predetermined narrative and glean what I could from my grandmother's horrific experience. My hope is that this story challenges you to consider that the truth could be different from what your eyes see and your ears hear as to that beloved stranger standing before you.

I dared to believe it could be different.

Prologue

November 2014

Nothing is really ever lost to us as long as we remember it.
L. M. Montgomery

Blind-sided by the news I'd been given moments earlier, I left the memory care center and slowly walked to my truck. My head pounded as I dug through the clutter in my purse, searching for my keys ... always searching for keys. Did I leave them inside again? Was I losing my mind? I couldn't go back in and face my mom, not after fleeing in tears.

Locating the keys under my pocketbook, I unlocked the door and climbed into the driver's seat. My head fell back as the soft leather embraced me. At least something felt good. Closing my eyes, I remembered the many times during our journey when I wanted to flee from the cruelty of Alzheimer's, and this moment was no exception. With just four weeks' notice that Mom would have to move, my thoughts centered on where she would now be spending Christmas. I had been given a month to uproot her from this community she'd considered home for more than three years and the familiar dwelling that had comforted her in late-stage Alzheimer's. The place where I thought she would live out her story—our story—to the end and the sequel to another that began with her mother, Ma.

※ ※ ※

It was mid-afternoon when the meeting ended, leaving me only a few hours to make calls. I stared at the phone in my hands, not knowing where to begin. Who in the world would take a late-stage Alzheimer's patient that another memory care center was throwing out? My dad's face appeared in my mind as his wise words came back to haunt me: "get it in writing." He wasn't referring to this situation but legal contracts in general. Three years ago, I could have used his guidance, but he'd been gone for the past twenty years.

I'd been cavalier as I filled out the paperwork to admit Mom, nonchalantly inquiring as to whether or not she could live out her life there. I thought I'd made it clear how important it was that I not have to move her again as I flipped page by page through the lengthy contract, most of which would have taken a JD to understand. It was the sales director, I believe, who'd assured me that most residents eventually died under the care of Hospice at this facility. *Most* was the operative word I'd failed to consider because at the time I had a more pressing concern on my mind: figuring out how I was going to convince Mom to move in.

November 2014

As I sat in my truck, crushed by the latest Alzheimer's punch to the gut, I looked up to Mom's room on the third floor. Remembering that only minutes ago, behind that glass, I spoke words to her that I never wanted to utter—one of the most painful conversations to have with a loved one. That big picture window now appeared black, but I laughed mockingly at the coincidence. Fully aware the effect was due to more light going in than coming out—a result of the sun's precise angle on that cold November day—the metaphor of a dark window caught me. I couldn't see through the mess just dropped in my lap, but, as I continued to stare up at the glass, black became the perfect backdrop for the video that launched in my mind.

Christmas music was blaring as my husband and brothers unpacked boxes of ornaments, trying to keep up with my sisters-in-law who were placing them on the tree. It was the week before Thanksgiving, the one holiday when Mom's family from locales north and south of Georgia descended upon our home in Atlanta for a bountiful feast and lots of merry making. It was also the week when we all visited Mom's nearby retirement community, in full-on celebration mode, to decorate her room for Christmas. Without a doubt, Christmas was Mom's favorite holiday.

I was removing sheets of packing paper from a bin and uncovering Christmas treasures when I pulled out a favorite of Mom's that doubled as a soothing nightlight: a cheerful, eighteen-inch snowman fitted with LED lights that slowly transitioned from red to green to blue. I placed it on the windowsill next to her bed, knowing it would spread warm light inside her room as darkness fell.

Decked out in a white turtleneck under a red sweater vest embroidered with dancing Santas, and a string of large, colorful Christmas bulbs draped around her neck, Mom flitted around in true form, placing Santa figurines on the credenza and randomly pulling one of the boys away from decorating to dance. Gleefully participating in a well-loved tradition that dated back to her childhood, she displayed a comfortable intimacy with this group even though she was no longer able to recall most of their names.

Travelling beyond that memory, I found myself in a crowd of well-dressed people surrounding a blackjack table. Alongside me were Mom and my husband Steve, as well as my brother Kevin and his wife Cathy. A dealer decked out in a black tuxedo was flipping one card over at a time before his croupier collected or paid out on bets placed. Surrounding us were round tables covered in black linen cloths with large plastic dice decorating the center. Black, red, and gold balloons fastened to the dice floated above the tables and around the doors. Neon blue and red lights highlighted the walls, and buffet tables loaded with appetizers and mouthwatering desserts were strategically placed. Residents of the retirement community and their families were spread across the two massive rooms beautifully transformed into a casino, trying their luck at poker, roulette, and craps.

The game moved fast and was exciting to watch, but Mom was impatient to move from an activity she no longer understood to an activity she'd never forgotten. I noticed her swaying to the rhythm as the band warmed up. Watching Mom move to instrumentals and lyrics, I realized she felt music, an experience called frisson, in which the brain releases dopamine, sending waves of pleasure throughout the body, or even chills.

Her steps were perfectly choregraphed to the music, and even in her mid-eighties, she still had the moves of Ginger Rogers. The casino dance floor was enticingly close, calling to her from some place in the innermost recesses of her brain. It was there, where some lucky memories remained safe from the damaging effects of beta-amyloid plaque or the mid-life small strokes that are part and parcel to some dementias, that Mom could return to the year 1945. Dancing with her girlfriends under the stars at the popular Ault Park in Cincinnati, she swung to the sounds of Duke Ellington and Benny Goodman. It didn't matter that most of the men were off fighting in World War II; those warm summer nights with her cousins and girlfriends were some of the fondest memories she had.

The next memory of mine placed me alongside some of my sisters-in-law who were in town visiting Mom. Standing next to each other, our eyes widened in amazement as we shook our heads from side to side, exchanging knowing glances at the situation about to unfold. What started out as a relaxing Saturday afternoon in the common area for these unsuspecting assisted-living residents erupted into a full-blown dance party with Mom and my brothers leading the way. Mom started the shenanigans by getting up to dance after hearing a song on the radio that stirred her into motion. Always ready to join the fun, my brothers shot into action, launching their rendition of E.U.'s "Da Butt," affectionately known by our family as the "Biggs Boys'

Butt Wiggle." Soon the reading glasses came off, books were put down, and attention diverted from the TV. A resident named Morrie jumped up, closely followed by a few others who, either alone or with help, joined in the dancing. Several staff members watched and laughed at this impromptu party and the fun their charges were having on an otherwise mundane afternoon.

Scenes like these and others flashed before me, one after another, until someone pulled their car in the spot next to mine, jolting me back to reality. Tears returned, and my shoulders slumped. My head collapsed onto the steering wheel as those happy memories faded and the unthinkable conversation I'd just had resurfaced, an unmistakable prompt to pull myself together, dry my eyes, and get after it.

⁂

Generations of Alzheimer's runs through my blood. Right now, I carry a lifetime of Christmases and other remembrances within me, hidden and stored somewhere deep within my brain. I think it's safe to say that on this plane of existence I am a compilation of my stored memories, but who am I if I lose access to them? What if the footbridge to all my lifetime experiences, along with the individuals included, becomes so damaged that I am blocked from remembering who I am and who they are?

I witnessed my grandmother and then my mom struggle with and eventually lose nearly all memory after Alzheimer's. Hard as it was to watch, their blank or frustrated expressions, often appearing before an incorrect or inappropriate response and sometimes preceding no response at all, intrigued me. Were they as troubled as I was by their inability to connect a name to a person or feelings to expressed thoughts? Did they feel abandoned, as I certainly would, by a process that normally allows us to transmit thoughts and feelings? Guessing from their irrational behaviors at times, I would say, yes, as the inability to communicate effectively can bring out the worst in everyone, from toddlers to the aged. I couldn't prove this, not scientifically, but I've experienced the frustration of being unable to adequately articulate thoughts, and I've seen the same struggle in my kids when they were younger manifested in tantrums or outbursts of anger.

Having done my research, I did understand a lot of the science behind Mom's failing brain, but what, if anything, of her would remain beyond the damage wasn't as clear. The immateriality of a soul can't be viewed on a CT scan, a fact that opens the door to much mystery and debate. Neuroscientists claim they can assign all attributes of the soul to different areas of the brain. If that's to be believed, it elicits the question, what purpose does a soul serve? Adding to the uncertainty is the camp of those who have faith in the presence of a soul but believe it departs after Alzheimer's, well before the body dies. That made no sense to me, but I'll admit after watching my grandmother disappear early in Alzheimer's, I wasn't sure what I believed.

What I knew was that if there was a possibility that Mom's life-force was gridlocked behind a chaotic brain network, I wasn't going to waste time philosophizing about the issue. I had to assume she was in there, trapped by the very means that allow me to express these thoughts in writing and for readers to understand them. To grasp her inner world, I had to slip into her skin, so to speak. My prior experience and knowledge of Alzheimer's was useless unless I pierced her confusion and operated—at least conceptually—from that space.

I imagined myself with Alzheimer's as I lay next to Steve in bed. Then switching to Mom's bewildered lens, I watched the individual sleeping next to me, and a warmth flowed through me. I felt so safe with him. Although I couldn't remember his name or who he was, I somehow knew him. I began to move toward him, but there were missing sections of the bridge between us, and I was stopped. Other people showed up as well, just beyond that gap, some big and some small. They called me Mom, Mumski, or Nina, Mare, Mary, and Marianne. How could I be so many different people? I smiled, as seeing them made me feel so good and I wanted to be with them, but I had no idea why.

Frightened by the fog that had descended on me—the reality of Mom's world—I wanted to flee, to get as far from that unknown and uncomfortable realm as I could, but only by remaining in that space could I feel her pain. Even on a minuscule scale, forcing myself to imagine that anguish helped me think and feel what she was likely thinking and feeling. That wasn't an easy position to hold, especially in the heat of difficult moments with her where I often failed miserably. I practiced this contemplative exercise when Mom lived with me, in the quiet early morning before I confronted her fury. When I put myself in her shoes, the door for empathy opened and my responses to her continual verbal confrontations grew much calmer.

⁂

As I write these pages, my eyes fall on my dog lying peacefully at my feet. I can name him, and the powerful feeling I have for him: it's called love, and his name is Charlie. Would my feelings for this beautiful animal change if I couldn't organize my thoughts and verbalize those words? Likewise, as I pass a mirror, I'm sometimes caught off guard by the reflected image. I still feel the same on the inside, but the mirror tells a different story. Does that make me not me? There were times in moderate Alzheimer's, mostly moments but sometimes hours, when Mom exhibited mystifying cognition that came out of nowhere. Within the span of those occurrences were extremes of emotions ranging from astonishment to grief. My mind could barely grasp the reality of having her back before she would disappear. However short or long, my awe and wonder in those backward movements of time drove me to question the reasons behind them.

Were these episodes when Mom suddenly remembered me and her life lived before Alzheimer's indicating that her memory was only a neuron's reconnection away? If it's all about cell death and wiring, is memory only a neurological function as some experts believe? Or, do our souls house our memories, while our brains serve as the complex processors that allow our inner selves to communicate in this world?

These questions had nudged me to different degrees since my grandmother's diagnosis, and the nudges became a full-blown shove after Mom's. The thought of another loved one's feelings and words, their life or being as I knew it, possibly trapped behind sticky plaque in their brain was a game changer for me. And the awful image of Mom's feisty spirit forever silenced in a mental prison awakened another, long-since muted voice. It was my grandmother's unsung story that gave me all the reasons I needed to unravel the mystery.

Chapter One

Where It All Began

Circa 1980

The end is in the beginning and lies far ahead.
Ralph Ellison

I was introduced to Alzheimer's when my grandmother, whom we called Ma, was diagnosed around 1980. She soon moved in with my family, and when her behaviors became too difficult to manage she went to a nursing home. Mom's original intention was to keep my grandmother in our family home forever, but that proved impossible. Sad as it was, her departure set the stage for the rest of this story.

We last saw Ma just after she entered the nursing home. This wasn't because we didn't visit—we did, regularly—but rather the consequence of a rapid downward spiral. The Ma we knew disappeared into a confused and apathetic stupor characteristic of someone over-medicated on anti-psychotics or suffering from late-stage Alzheimer's. But she wasn't anywhere near late stage. Her lethargy came on virtually overnight, and Mom spent the following decade in a futile attempt to bring her mother back, to reestablish some of the mother-daughter relationship that was lost, but it was, tragically, gone for good.

That failure was devastating but pivotal in how life played out for my mother. Decades after my grandmother passed, careful exploration of her journey acted as a *Sankofa*, a term used by the Akan tribe in Ghana who believe the past is a useful and powerful guide for influencing the future. Ma's journey would have meant nothing more than a miserable chapter in our family's history if the lingering wisdom hidden in her struggles died with her.

Losing Ma in that awful way haunted Mom for the rest of her life—an open wound that never healed. Her phobia then became mine. Twenty years later that fear became a reality, but this time Alzheimer's introduced itself in a very different and veiled form than previously experienced. Mom morphed into Debby Downer as she became overly sensitive and critical of others. Her growing paranoia caused her to accuse family members and friends of ridiculous offenses. Alzheimer's was quietly stalking her, creeping through the cellar door and operating in the dark backrooms of her brain. This biological warfare began years before we noticed anything unusual, as Alzheimer's is known to begin in the brain decades before the first clinical symptoms appear.

After Mom was diagnosed, I vowed to leave no stone unturned in keeping her from the abyss that claimed my grandmother. I had to be her advocate, so I schooled myself in the disease, starting with the Alzheimer's Association's website and its research links. I participated in online forums with caregivers sharing information and coping skills and joined local Alzheimer's support groups. I grilled health care professionals, followed Alzheimer's blogs, and read countless books on Alzheimer's and dementia. I filled my brain with everything I could find while Mom's brain was slowly leaking out her precious memories.

Although many of the books were educational and inspirational, especially stories of the selfless spirits of caregivers, the central message remained: your loved one will die while still living. I'd already lived that narrative with Ma, and while I understood that the mother I knew—and who knew me—would change irretrievably, I needed a different perspective. I wanted more for Mom and for myself. I wanted her to remain alive in her spirit, however that might look, until her physical body gave way to the earth.

Part of me always yearned to bring Mom back, and to return to the days before her diagnosis, but there was—and is—no cure. I often lingered on the threshold of these two worlds—the before and the after—but ruminating on what used to be simply served as a depressant that kept me from moving forward. I believed I'd been entrusted with this task of ushering Mom through this new door, much in the same way God trusted me with my kids and their journeys toward independence. My job was clear: to keep Mom from disappearing. Unlike my grandmother, Mom was not going to slip through my fingers.

The average life expectancy for one with late onset Alzheimer's is eight-to-ten years but varies with the type of dementia, overall health, and age at diagnosis. I wanted to make the most of those years. I had many questions for Mom's doctors over the course of her journey, some they couldn't or wouldn't answer because they fell beyond the scope of traditional medicine. Questions like: "Does my mom exist beyond her brain damage?" or "Is she still in there, somewhere?" were usually received with a kind but often patronizing smile followed by an unequivocally clinical answer referencing beta-amyloid plaque, tau tangles, mini-strokes in midlife, and inflammation.

Piggybacked on that information came, "At the present time the damage to her brain is irreversible," followed by, "Here is the approximate timeline for dementia, so I would recommend that you make plans for her future care because soon she will not have the capacity to do so." That's sound advice for any life-altering, and eventually life-ending, disease like Alzheimer's, and I understood the importance of managing those details. The answer I sought, however, existed beyond the medical diagnosis and annals of scientific journals. Fortunately, over the course of Mom's diagnosed journey, I did find practitioners who understood and respected my question and were willing to delve into that mystery with me.

I fully accepted there wasn't a drug to bring her back, but what I didn't accept was that "no medical cure" was the only remedy offered. Wasn't there another path to healing? Since allopathic medicine offered no hope, I knew that my optimism for any type of life that held value for Mom would come up against her mental decline, which was slowly becoming more pronounced. I didn't want to let her go, so I knew I had to disprove what many still believed: that Alzheimer's commandeers its victims, whisking them off to some distant land while leaving behind only their empty shell.

Ask anyone who knew Mom, and they will say she was a great dancer—always the first on the dance floor and the last one off. She danced her way through many of life's hardships, leading to a belief that a steely will could conquer anything. Would this also hold true for Alzheimer's? Was her staunch declaration to never submit (to anything, including this disease) powerful enough to overcome the physiological damage to her brain? In other words, could her kick-ass spirit shine through Alzheimer's?

I was fully aware and realistic—my mom had Alzheimer's. It was as if she was standing at the airport gate holding a boarding pass stamped "dementia," about to board a plane with no return ticket, headed in the same direction my grandmother had travelled. Meanwhile, I felt stuck in security, surrounded and hindered by voices that whispered, "She will soon become a vacant address." I knew that if there was any chance to prove that viewpoint wrong, I had to act fast. I had to meet her where she was in the progression of the disease and recognize her beyond the many identities she would eventually assume, outside of the mother she was to me. So, I jumped that security line and ran like hell, closely pursued by pounding feet and voices that screamed, "It doesn't work that way, you will never find her!"

CHAPTER TWO

This Thing Called Memory

> *How can we live out our lives?*
> *How will we know it's us without our past?*
> JOHN STEINBECK

My earliest memory dates to when I was three. I'm in my bed, which is next to the large window overlooking our front porch, where Mom is talking to Mrs. Springer, our neighbor across the cul-de-sac and her good friend. Because our home is not air-conditioned, the horizontal glass panels in the window frame are cranked out, letting in the cool night air. Having drifted off to sleep earlier, I am now awakened by the comforting melody of crickets and two familiar voices speaking in hushed tones. I don't hear their actual conversation, but the chirps of the crickets and the humdrum of the ladies' dialogue blends into a comforting cadence. Reassured that all is well in my world, I am lulled back to sleep.

Another memory surfaces—young children playing in a school yard—and I flash back to kindergarten. Sitting at my desk, I lean forward, squeezing my crossed legs together as tightly as I can. Although I remember my teacher as very kind, I'm terrified of asking permission to use the bathroom. I don't ask, thus wetting my panties.

Hiking with my husband, Steve, and our family along rocky creek beds brings back recollections of long childhood summer days with my brothers, playing in the creek that ran behind our house. The video that launches this time is of us jumping from rock to rock, searching out crawfish. Finding them burrowed in the wet mud below the rocks, we carefully pick them up by their midsections as the larger ones pack a powerful pinch.

Still more memories from my childhood pop up when I look to the sky on a clear night and recall the little green pup tents dotting my backyard. Lying on our backs in the cool grass, my brothers and I stare at the sky as the dwindling light of day disappears and the first evening stars flicker into view. Our eyes then turn toward our second-story windows, eagerly anticipating the final lamp to dowse in our parents' bedroom. Confident they're down for the count, we sneak off to King Kwik, a local convenience store. Hands full of candy and Icees, we rush home with our treats before anyone notices we're gone.

These are just some of my long-term memories, and they are episodic, which means I lived them with specific individuals in a certain time and place. Whenever I recall this type of memory, the associated emotions also travel with them. These recollections may be imperfect because they are influenced by many factors such as our perception of the event when it happened, and our emotional response to it. Because personal views of a situation are subjective, two individuals witnessing the same event may later recall different things. According to an article in *healthline,* "Emotions serve as subjective reactions to objective events."[6] Perfect or imperfect, memories that I do recall from my childhood, and beyond, all contribute to the mosaic of who I am today: daughter, sister, wife, mother, grandmother, and friend.

While I constantly make more memories, and some experts say we create as many as seventy-four gigabytes of potential memories a day, most of what we generate is useless. If our brains tried to hold everything we experience, see, and hear in a day, they would overload with unessential information, and, like a computer, crash. Memories we do retain, especially if attached to strong emotions, are captured by a process that occurs within a healthy, functioning brain.

※ ※ ※

Presently, I am aware of who I am, what past events have shaped me, and how I arrived at this moment and place in time. I know these things because my brain is working properly; the neurons inside are talking with each other then communicating back to me. Before Alzheimer's, I took this phenomenon for granted—

this intricate collaboration of processes allowing me to recall the important things that have happened up until this moment to successfully live in the next.

Webster's dictionary defines *memory* as "the power or process of reproducing or recalling what has been learned and retained, especially through associative mechanisms; a particular act of recall or recollection; an image or impression of one that is remembered; or the time within which past events can be or are remembered." But that definition is an underestimation of the miracle occurring when the process of memory performs properly. Within its mere six letters, the entirety of my human existence to date is held, creating the unique individual I have become. The ability to recall a memory is crucial, for without it I might be a drifter in an alien land, unable to recognize—or at least verbalize—who those are surrounding me, understand their language, or operate in an independent state. Eventually, I may even forget the vital functions allowing my physical organism to continue walking, talking, breathing, and swallowing.

Memories my brain deems important enough to be stored are greeted by the secretary sitting at my frontal lobe. After checking them in, she delivers and records them in the hippocampus, located in the medial (middle) brain lobes. Once admitted, they are sent out to numerous warehouses within the cortical area, the brain's gray, wrinkly, outer layer. They are filed there in cabinets until I retrieve them. Often a cue from my environment in the form of something seen, heard, smelled, or tasted conjures up that stored memory. Then through a complicated but quick retrieval process, I am escorted back to that time, event, or person.

For example, whenever I hear the song "Dust in the Wind," I am transported back to the year 1978. It is spring break, and I am camping on a beach at Fort De Soto State Park, Florida. Classmates from our advanced biology class, along with a few teachers from Mother of Mercy High School in Cincinnati, Ohio, made the long trip south to study the ecosystem of coastal waters. Lying on a towel alongside my peers, I see the blazing sun in the cloudless blue sky, hear the rich instrumentals and wistful lyrics of Kansas reminding me of the fleeting nature of our lives, and feel the previous day's blistering sunburn on the tops of my feet.

That's the simple explanation of how we remember. When the hippocampus is damaged, however, the experience happens but the secretary never records it. The incoming memory does a fly-by right over the hippocampus and vaporizes as if it never existed.

Poof, it's gone.

This is what happens with short-term memory loss in Alzheimer's and other types of dementia. It explains the adage often applied to Alzheimer's disease: "last in, first out; first in, last out." Long-term implicit memories, including procedural ones that tell us how to do things, have been stored in our brains since childhood. The ability to brush our teeth, pour cereal into a bowl, and even play the piano is largely unconscious because those activities became muscle memory in our brains through years of repetition.

If Mom could have balanced herself on a bike in moderate dementia, her body would have remembered how to turn the pedals and move the bike forward even as she looked at me running alongside of her, clueless I was her daughter. These habitual, deep-seated repetitions are our "first in, last out" memories. More recent events, such as where the car is parked, the movie just seen, and where the car keys were left are the "last in, first out."

Short-term memory loss occurs because the "last in" experiences never get encoded. You don't remember having a conversation with your son five minutes ago, so you repeat it, again and again. Your daughter dropped you off at Dillard's department store, but your brain didn't record it. After a few hours of shopping, heaped with bags full of the latest fashion finds, you head out the door to find your car. Roaming the parking lot in a frenzied, fruitless search, you convince yourself and everyone around you that your car was stolen. When your daughter returns to the store's entrance at the agreed pickup time, she spots you sitting in a police car. Seeing you there terrifies her, but you're so busy chatting with the nice police officer and rooting through your purse for your keys that you don't notice. You've also forgotten the make, model, and color of your stolen vehicle.

Sometimes the effects of Alzheimer's are more subtle. You return from the market with bags of groceries in tow, and your keys—along with the frozen fish and ice cream—land in the freezer. Later, when the keys are not on their usual hook, you set out to find them, but on the way you get distracted. The dog is barking because the mailman delivered the mail, and you stop to retrieve it. Just then the dryer buzzer goes off, and you mindlessly drop the mail on a nearby chair as you head to the laundry room. Once there you start to fold clothes when your nose picks up the scent of something burning. Panicked, you rush to the kitchen where smoke is billowing up from the now waterless pot of carrots left on the stove. They are burned to the bottom of the pan. The keys, the real culprit behind this failed mission, are long forgotten. Perhaps most terrifying however, is the day that comes when you take those keys off the hook and stare down at them, desperately trying to remember what they're used for—or who they belong to.

When the brain is unable to register new memories, it's like ending up as Lucy in *50 First Dates*, living in a perpetual state of now. In some ways short-term memory loss is like having a dream you don't remember. An EEG records brain wave activity during REM sleep and documents that you were dreaming, but you have no memory of that dream. With Alzheimer's, you do and say things that others see and hear (and can remember), but you have no memory of these occurrences. The only thing you know is that your daughter or son infuriates you every time they say, "Mom, you just asked me that question," or "Mom, you told me that story three times in the last hour," or "Mom, why are your keys in the freezer?"

According to the National Institute on Aging, "Dementia is the loss of cognitive functioning—thinking, remembering, and reasoning—and behavioral abilities to such an extent that it interferes with a person's daily life and activities." Dementia is an umbrella term for many forms of this disease. Alzheimer's dementia is the most common, accounting for 60 to 80 percent of all diagnoses. Vascular dementia is second most common, followed in descending order by dementia with Lewy bodies, mixed dementia, Parkinson's dementia, frontotemporal dementia, and others. My mom and maternal grandmother were both diagnosed with Alzheimer's dementia, although I now believe that Mom's was more of a mixed dementia. Their diagnoses may have been the same, but their paths were vastly different.

Parents always hope to improve life for the next generation; wanting better experiences for their children in areas where they may have struggled. In this vein my grandmother served as Alzheimer's ambassador extraordinaire to this granddaughter, carrying many lessons from the previous age into the next. My mom hoped against hope, while caring for my grandmother, that there was still a life in Ma beyond her failing cognition, which was not evident during their prolonged journey. I honestly don't know how Mom would have fared under my care if Ma's painful experience hadn't been a pivotal point of reference for both of us as it represented everything that didn't work the first time.

Chapter Three

A Bit about Ma

(1899-1992)

*The world breaks everyone, and afterward,
some are strong at the broken places.*
Ernest Hemingway

Shortly after Ma was born in 1899—at the turn of a century that would usher in five wars for the US, the Great Depression, and major scientific advancements that radically changed how medicine is practiced—there was a young woman experiencing bizarre symptoms that would later become associated with what we now know as Alzheimer's. The doctor that followed her discovered, upon an autopsy of her brain, strange looking plaque formations. Despite his best intentions to bring these discoveries forward for further research, that plaque, which would later be recognized as the hallmark of this disease, remained in the notes of his files for almost three quarters of a century.[7] Sometime during the latter part of that period, and unbeknownst to my grandmother and her family, that same insidious intruder began setting up residence in Ma's brain.

My grandmother was a strong woman with a sturdy body and a healthy heart that pumped life-sustaining blood through her vessels well into her eighth decade. She exuded copious amounts of energy and stamina, and I can't remember her ever being sick. She possessed a sound mind, not overly educated, but in control and able to confront the challenges and obstacles life threw at her, which at times were many. Mostly though, she was extremely strong-willed, assertive, and determined—traits that continued in her daughter, my mom.

My grandfather died of a heart attack while Ma was still in her fifties, before I was born, and she lived independently and successfully for another two and a half decades. She never remarried or even considered another companion, her favorite response being, "I had one good man!"

※ ※ ※

Ma was a big presence in our family as I was growing up. My dad worked and was away for long hours, and Mom was employed part-time. During those gaps, my grandmother watched my five brothers and me, folding clothes, helping with meals, and trying to keep us all in line. Too many times I heard her say, "Your mother has a front row seat reserved for her in heaven!" I knew she was right, as the six of us were a pack of wolves disguised as humans!

A Bit about Ma

As I got older, I remember her travelling, often trekking alone to Las Vegas, which was unusual for a woman her age, further proving her tenacity. She was a gambler at heart and adored horse racing. Solo, she often made her way to River Downs racetrack, along the banks of the Ohio River, making several changes on the bus line before reaching her destination.

Alzheimer's came along in her late seventies. Prior to that she lived independently in a four-family apartment. Several days a week she walked the quarter mile to the shopping center where my mom still worked. Her first stop was Woolworth's Five-and-Ten, where she sat at the counter and ordered lunch before she spent the afternoon drifting in and out of the stores lining the Western Hills shopping center. Waiting for Mom to finish up, she landed on the bench outside of McAlpin's department store, taking in the afternoon sun.

She was a talker, and if you sat next to her, you would learn everything about her family, which was comprised of two daughters, one son, and seventeen grandchildren. The next thing out of her mouth was always to tell you that her son, Wally, was a doctor. She was so proud of him. She owned that bench in her loose-fitting comfortable house dress and some version of a patent leather, low-heeled shoe. Costume jewelry was draped at her neck and heavy earrings clipped to her lobes. Her short wig sat high on her forehead and gray glasses with pointed sides rested on her nose. She carried a black purse with a round handle that fit snugly in the crux of her elbow. You had to pass by quick or you'd find yourself unable to escape her chatty web.

It surprised us, then, when she got lost on her way to McAlpin's, ending up in nearby stores asking for her daughter. Someone from that store would call Mom's work and have her paged. She would then leave work, retrieve Ma, and drive her home. She was concerned Ma was becoming forgetful but attributed the confusion to normal aging or "senility" as it was often referred to. After all, there were no documented cases of Alzheimer's in Ma's family. No one knew much about it at all, so there was no reason to suspect anything other than age-related memory loss.

Not long after these incidents though, Ma began showing signs of paranoia. She started calling Mom at night to report strange noises outside her second-story apartment window. My parents would drive to her apartment and Dad would walk the perimeter of the building while Mom and Ma watched from her kitchen window. Coming back inside, Dad assured Ma everything was fine. The paranoia increased and soon she was waking my parents up at all hours of the night, describing "scary men" standing below her window looking up at her.

Her fear escalated until she became terrified to live alone. By then she was beginning to lose and misplace things. We found random items in strange places—hairspray in her refrigerator, melted ice cream in the oven. Mom's biggest fear was that Ma would forget to turn off the stove and burn the building down. It was clear she could no longer live by herself, and, because of financial limitations, home health care was not a viable option. Mom's only choices were a nursing home or moving Ma in with us. Since Mom wouldn't consider a nursing home, Ma moved in.

Chapter Four

She's Running Away

The Early Eighties

If ever I was running, it was towards you.
Jennifer Elizabeth

By the time I arrived on the planet, Ma had already lost a young child and her husband. She was a quiet survivor; growing up, I never observed her grief nor heard her speak of the loss. I knew the story only because it was recounted to me by my mom with the admonishment never to speak of it around Ma. What I observed from the sidelines as a grandchild who loved this large personality was a woman resilient to heartache. In my young mind, she demonstrated true grit in her ability to suppress painful memories. Later, I would come to see how silenced trauma became detrimental to her mental health.

Her loss resurfaced after Alzheimer's, and the anguish held in all those years over the death of her youngest came barreling back. Like many dementia sufferers, she began running away but always toward someone she never forgot. The umbilical cord that sustained this child in her womb may have been cut at birth, but the love between them was never severed.

※ ※ ※

"Where is Ma?"

I was lying on my bed reading when Mom burst through the door, eyes wide with fear as she scanned my room for evidence of my grandmother, who had managed once again to escape our home and disappear into the night. I jumped off the bed, threw on a coat, and joined the search, confident Ma was somewhere close by.

Ma began "taking off" shortly after she came to live with us. Present-day terminology would label her a "flight risk" or call her behavior "wandering."[8] She was in hot pursuit of a boy whose being was so intimately woven through her heart that even Alzheimer's couldn't erase him. This indestructible bond was with her youngest son, Donnie, who had died as a toddler. Most evenings around sundown, she'd become agitated and wander aimlessly throughout the house looking for him. The memory of him, lingering quietly in her subconscious most of her life, was now making a loud resurgence.

Now called "Sundowners Syndrome," this unusual activity is defined by the Mayo Clinic as a "state of confusion occurring in the late afternoon and lasting into the night." Sundowning "can cause different behaviors, such as confusion, anxiety, aggression or ignoring directions," and "can also lead to pacing or wandering."[9] Researchers have not yet discovered its cause and some link it to a disturbance in circadian rhythms, but there are many factors that may exacerbate the condition, as well as tips to reduce the potential for it.[10]

It was during the transition between daylight and darkness—as the earth continued its rotation around the sun, tilting slightly away from its source of heat and light—that Ma experienced increased confusion and restlessness. In her disordered state of mind, a memory flickered and perhaps ignited ensuing anxiety with a reenactment of the day she lost her son. I don't know what fanned those flames, but I do know my grandmother responded the way any mother would if their child was missing—she stopped at nothing to find him.

The heartbreaking echoes of her desperate search resonated throughout our home, night after night.

"Where is my baby, where is my baby?" she wailed, darting from room to room.

Mom often asked her, "What baby, Mother?" and she would respond, "Donnie, my baby Donnie."

She was a formidable force as she assumed the bearing of a rescue dog tracking down a scent, embarking on that search with total and reckless abandon. Nothing else mattered, and no amount of reasoning could redirect her when caught in the throes of that awful memory. So, after many unsuccessful attempts to divert her, we found it best to let her search, which she sometimes did for hours.

My parents were still living in their modest, yellow-brick home that sat back from the wide circle on Highfields Lane on the west side of Cincinnati. The backyard was large, bordered by a tree-lined creek bed that swelled into a raging river after heavy rains, but it always held water. Beyond the creek and up the hill was another neighborhood, and, in the winter, you could see through the bare trees to the backs of those homes. It was a steep climb up, and I often traversed it on my walk to school and ended up on my butt coming home if the slope was icy or wet. Sledding down that hill was exciting if you could steer clear of the trees and stop before you hit the creek. That didn't always happen, as my brother Tim can attest.

My parents built that house when they were expecting their fourth son, my brother Joe. Two additional kids later, their three-bedroom, one-and-one-half-bath home began bursting at the seams. My dad finished the walkout level with an additional family room, bedroom, and bathroom. There was also a second-story deck off the back, as the front of the house was built into an elevation. The covered front porch faced the circle. That's often where my grandmother would be on warm afternoons, rocking, and watching the kids play games in the street—until she began wandering off.

This wasn't Ma's first breakout, and our neighbors were accustomed to both looking for and looking out for her. If speed dial had existed then, the local police would have been first on the list. My parents had reconfigured the locks and were confident their home was escape-proof, but this incident left them dumbfounded. In hindsight, it's easy to understand what Ma pulled off that night as mothers throughout history have achieved mind-boggling feats on behalf of their children.

On that evening, my grandmother left her bedroom in the back of the house, slipping by all of us on the main level as she made her way down the steep steps to the walkout level below. Once there, she dragged a heavy chair from the family room to the door. Then, stepping her hefty, eighty-year-old body onto the chair, she succeeded in sliding the cylindrical door bolt horizontally through its tight encasement—a challenge for everyone in our family—and out she went.

The police were notified and the search and rescue was well underway when a call came in. Ma had been found by a resident in the neighborhood up the hill behind my parents' home. The police were on their way to pick her up and bring her back. My grandmother was safe, and we all breathed a collective sigh of relief, but Mom just lowered her head into her hands. She was weary from trying to keep ahead of Ma's disease and shielding her from harm, an exhaustion further exacerbated by lack of sleep. Like the rest of us, she was shocked that Ma had not only escaped our home but also accessed the neighborhood behind and above us, barefoot and thinly clad on a cold, dark night.

In retrospect, I have no doubt my grandmother encountered, night after night, the same gut-wrenching terror I experienced one summer afternoon when my three-year-old son, Brady, went missing. We were visiting my mom and dad, and Brady was sitting in front of my parents' console TV in the same basement family room from which Ma had escaped. He was playing with his action figures while watching the movie, *Teenage Mutant Ninja Turtles*. That's where I left him while Mom and I walked outside to talk to our neighbor over the fence. I felt comfortable leaving him there as Dad was only a few steps away in the back bedroom, talking on his ham radio. When Mom and I came back inside, Brady and our dog Maggie were gone.

Memories of my grandmother's wild searches for her son quickly resurfaced in me as we combed the house, the yard, and the cul-de-sac. Frantic, I ran up the street with Dad following me in his car. Scanning yards as I ran, I screamed, "Brady! Brady!" asking any neighbors outside if they had seen a small blond boy with a little white dog.

My grandmother ran from room to room, opening closet doors and getting down on her knees to look under the beds. She wailed, "Where is my baby, where is my baby?"

Approaching the end of my parents' street, I looked right to the next intersection where traffic was at a standstill. Arriving at that junction and looking up the hill, I gasped at the sight of flashing red lights in the very direction a neighbor reported seeing a little boy and his dog. I brushed off my panic and then experienced a fleeting sensation of annoyance at this guy for not stopping a toddler walking alone on a busy street. I ran on.

Breathing heavily, my grandmother held tightly to the rail as she lumbered down the basement steps and hurried toward the door. She twisted the doorknob, but it was locked from above. Lugging a large chair from the TV room, she stepped up onto it and yanked at the deadbolt, but it didn't budge. She tried again and again, desperately twisting, pushing, and pulling on that stubborn bolt until finally it slid free. Getting down, she shoved the chair away, flung open the door, and entered the cold, black night.

I was beside myself as myriad irrational thoughts blew up in my brain like the grand finale of a fireworks display: The dog pulled him into the street, he tried to cross the street but didn't look both ways, a car ran off the road and hit him. Growing up, one of my dogs was hit by a car and killed on this street, and I was now certain Brady had suffered the same fate. Dread, that crippling foreboding of the worst possible scenario, wrapped its fingers around my heart and squeezed, making it difficult to breathe as I ran. My mind foresaw my sweet child lying in a blood-soaked heap with emergency personnel kneeling by his side, desperately trying to save his young life.

Outside, Ma's eyes slowly adjusted to the darkness. Rubbing her upper arms while shivering from the cold, she wondered which way to go. She was angry no one would help find him. He was only three. Did he even have a coat on? Surely, he would get lost or an animal would attack him. Even worse, someone would take him, and she would never see him again. She felt her heart pounding through her chest as her breathing became short and labored. Off in the distance she saw a light.

I had to get to Brady but was terrified of how I might find him. My mind froze, but my body kept moving. I don't remember my feet hitting the pavement as I ran the quarter mile toward the accident, but they propelled me at warp speed. I flew toward those flashing red lights, the same spot where a young boy I knew growing up lost his life darting across that heavily travelled road. He was trying to get to his uncle parked on the other side. A blanket of fear enveloped me, but at the same time an instinctive, feral impulse emerged from the depths of my being and ripped through my body, overpowering me, prodding me forward. This unrestricted force had no limits, and I knew in that instant I would break through a brick wall to reach my son.

Ma felt something cutting into her feet as she stumbled across rocks, falling several times in the water before reaching the other side. Scrambling through prickly bushes, she pushed away the branches scratching her face and arms. She began to climb, falling on all fours as her cumbersome body resisted the steep ascent.

"Where is my baby, where is my baby?" she cried aloud in the darkness as she crawled over the frozen earth, slowly inching her way toward the light at the top of the hill. He was cold and alone, and nothing, absolutely nothing would stop her from finding him.

Whenever I recall my search for Brady, the panic and fear I felt on that day can still well up. An experience of that magnitude, regardless of the ending, is a trauma that resides permanently within. The amygdala, an almond-shaped structure located in the region of the brain behind the ears–also known as the "fight or flight" center–plays a significant role in how highly emotional experiences influence memory. "As we go about our lives, we experience a variety of events, most of which we forget. By contrast, we tend to form long lasting and vivid memories for emotionally arousing or stressful events."[11] These intense memories are attached to powerful, deep-seated emotions that leave lasting imprints on our psyche. The amygdala is affected to varying degrees in early Alzheimer's disease.

Usually when I hear of a child gone missing or I can't immediately find a grandchild in my home, that memory surfaces and an irrational panic sets in. Running a close second to that terrifying recollection is another, and, when it overtakes and passes the first, I remember the immense sense of relief as I shoved my way through the throng of bystanders and spied a tiny speck of blond hair. Brady was hidden in the towering crowd, standing innocently beside our little white dog, holding the hand of a police officer. He'd been so absorbed by the unfolding display of flashing lights and activity of first responders tending to the injured from an accident he'd witnessed, he never heard me screaming his name.

※ ※ ※

Half a century after my grandmother lost her youngest, she experienced—almost nightly—a similar resurfacing of this life-changing tragedy compliments of her amygdala. But unlike my situation, her memory couldn't pull up the rest of the story. She was allowed no closure, and no amount of reasoning could convince Ma that Donnie was no longer missing, so she searched and searched and searched.

Despite her damaged brain, Donnie dwelled within Ma. The grief over his loss lingered in a space we couldn't touch or see with human eyes or brain scans or blood work. Nevertheless, it endured, and I look to my grandmother and her mental anguish during those searches as evidence of its ongoing presence. Many scenarios may have played out in her mind as she searched, but, in the end, her ability to overcome countless deterrents was fueled by the same maternal love as mine—a love that doesn't live in the brain, transcends the grasp of time, and powerfully defies the hurricane force winds of disease.

Alzheimer's set up a scenario in Ma's brain where she couldn't function without the help of others, remember her last conversation, or tell the names of her grandchildren. But she remembered her youngest son, and at that intersection where the past collided with the present, the 1930s returned and Donnie was gone.

Thankfully, Ma would eventually grow weary after her searches and give in to sleep, but Donnie reemerged night after night, and the running resumed. Breaking through the damage of her unrelentingly broken brain that couldn't remember was an equally unrelenting broken heart that couldn't forget.

Chapter Five

The Entertaining Moments of Alzheimer's

The Early Eighties

There is a fine line that separates laughter and pain, comedy and tragedy, humor and hurt.
Erma Bombeck

As teenagers without the burden and responsibilities of caregiving, my brother and I found a lot of Ma's behaviors funny. Not so for Mom though as she saw her mission not just to keep Ma safe but also to somehow—against all odds—bring her back from the grip of Alzheimer's. Although she never verbalized it, I could see by Mom's caregiving approach that my grandmother was becoming her child.

I was in my late teens when Ma was diagnosed, and, like everyone else, I didn't understand this disease. I wanted my grandmother to act like my grandmother, but at the same time I sensed a vulnerability that was out of character for her because her normal demeanor was confident and saucy. Mom recognized this too, and that was her greatest conflict as she vacillated between trying to preserve my grandmother in the crumbling reality that was her mother and accepting the emerging reality that her mother was regressing into a childlike dependent. Mom couldn't make sense of this mysterious disease, and out of frustration tried to return Ma to the real world each time she repeated herself or told a tall tale. My grandmother's contrived stories were highly entertaining and usually based on a fact or current event she had seen on TV, heard on the radio, or overheard from someone else. She then imbedded herself into that narrative and skillfully spun it into a fantastic (but imaginary) memory she recalled in vivid detail.

My mom, after her diagnosis, shared similar awe-inspiring life adventures. For example, she once jumped out of a plane at ten thousand feet, falling alongside President George H. W. Bush as he celebrated his eightieth birthday—both parachuting safely to the ground. On another occasion she shared a delicious luncheon with First Lady Barbara Bush on the Bushes' veranda. They feasted on fresh fish, overlooking the vast and endless expanse of brilliant blue ocean at the Bushes' home in Kennebunkport, Maine. Mom then raced that beautiful and electrifying chestnut stallion, Secretariat, to its first-place finish at the Kentucky Derby. In addition, she and my dad attended a Super Bowl game sitting right behind the Cincinnati Bengals' bench on the fifty-yard line, "so close," she would say, that she could almost touch the players (which to our knowledge never happened). Most impressive, though, is the story of Mom surviving her ocean liner's devastating collision with an iceberg aboard the *Titanic* in April 1912, thirteen years before she was born.

Both Ma and Mom lived exciting and adventurous lives in this otherworldly "dementia dimension," their new memories giving them much pleasure as they boasted about these escapades. They genuinely believed these accounts however outrageous they sounded to all of us. Fictitious tales? Yes. But we oohed and aahed at Mom's "memorable memories," allowing her to dwell in those moments, even encouraging her with questions surrounding the experiences. This was in stark contrast to our hushed responses to Ma's stories because we had learned the first time around that she had no control over those tall tales.

"Confabulation is a neuropsychiatric disorder wherein a patient generates a false memory without the intention of deceit. The patient believes the statement to be truthful, hence the descriptive term 'honest lying.'"[12] It occurs in early Alzheimer's, and, although researchers have not conclusively identified the neural pathways involved in the process, it most likely begins like every other memory process with a cue that initiates the route. That cue then hits a glitch on its path to retrieve the memory, causing some of if not all the details to be inaccurate. The events that Mom and Ma described were real and many of the details were accurate; the inaccuracy was their part in the narrative.

My brother Kevin and I were the last of the six kids still living at home when my grandmother lived with us. During that time, early on in her disease, she would regale us with her outlandish stories. Kevin and I would crack up, aware they were fabricated yet still finding them hilarious. My grandmother would light up at the positive attention and carry on. Mom was never amused and would instruct us to keep Ma in the present. She was losing her and believed, at least early on, my grandmother might exercise some control over her strange behaviors. Perhaps calling her out would somehow rescue her from the clutches of this monster.

I understood Mom thinking she could bring Ma back, because Ma's memory was so inconsistent. She would carry on a normal conversation in one sitting, remembering she went to Shillito's department store with Mom during the day then forget how to set the dinner table at night. In the early eighties, education and access to information surrounding Alzheimer's was so limited that we were as confused as Ma. It was the blind leading the blind.

While Ma lived with us, I was dating Steve, who had become a best friend to Kevin. The three of us would often sit around the kitchen table playing cards with my grandmother after dinner. When it got late and we wanted to move on to something else, we would tell her it was time to turn in, but she would stubbornly refuse to get up. Wagging her finger at Steve and Kevin she would boldly state, "I am not going anywhere until you boys go home!"

She couldn't remember that Kevin was her grandson, but she knew full well that a young girl should not be left alone with two boys, especially at night. My brother would protest, teasing Ma that he was not only my brother, but also her grandson. "Ma!

I live here!" Not to be deterred, she'd defiantly cross her arms and stand her ground until both got up and pretended to leave the house. Then, in a motherly fashion, she would lecture me about the dangers of having boys hanging around the house after dark. We were looking after our grandmother in her declining mental state, but she watched over me with a protective maternal instinct that defied her disease.

Like the rest of our family, my grandmother had a sweet tooth, and it's doubtful many days passed without her indulging in her favorite dessert. Although she loved all sweets, her foremost passion was ice cream—any flavor. I can attest to the fact that it's hard to grow up in Cincinnati, home to Graeter's and United Dairy Farmers, without developing a serious addiction to the stuff. My grandmother was always ready with her change purse in the pocket of her dress, pouncing on any unsuspecting victim who entered our home, asking sweetly for a ride to the ice cream parlor.

Unfortunately, her Type 2 diabetes necessitated restrictions on how much she could eat. Mom would buy a few cartons of ice cream during her weekly shopping trip to the market only to find them all consumed a few days later. Of course, my grandmother denied this because in truth she couldn't remember, and any spoon or bowl had been wiped off and placed neatly back in the cabinet or drawer, dirty. That created another issue.

When a carton of ice cream went missing, and after making sure neither my brother nor I had indulged a late-night craving, Mom would question my grandmother. Ma would appear so sweet and naive as she sat at our wooden kitchen table, looking as surprised as a child caught with her hand in the cookie jar. She would staunchly refute the claim that she ate the entire carton of ice cream, even as telltale chocolate stains dotted the front of her blouse.

Her eyes would widen as she stared at my mom, incredulous at being accused of such a wrongdoing, as she innocently stated in a small voice, "I didn't even know we *had* ice cream." We didn't have the sugar-free alternatives available to us, so Mom was left with two options: rid the house of ice cream (which would not have gone over well with the rest of the family) or padlock the fridge. The latter solution made sense not only because of the ice cream but also because my grandmother didn't know when to stop eating, especially sweets.

For years, researchers have stressed the link between Type 2 diabetes and dementias, but newer studies point with concern to blood glucose levels in what they refer to as the fasting-prediabetic range of 100-126. An article in the *Harvard Health Blog* cites a study in the *New England Journal of Medicine* where study author Dr. David Nathan, a Harvard Medical School professor and the director of the Diabetes Center and Clinical Research Center at Massachusetts General Hospital, demonstrates that individuals without diabetes but with elevated blood sugar levels increase their risk of dementia. "It establishes for the first time, convincingly, that there is a link between dementia and elevated blood sugars in the non-diabetic range."[13]

My parents installed a combination padlock on their refrigerator as a last resort to control my grandmother's diabetes, which understandably infuriated Ma. She couldn't grasp the dangers of diabetes or how her lifetime indulgence in a dairy product she loved could be bad for her, but that didn't stop my mom from continually explaining it. I heard that conversation at least once a day as they danced in circles around the subject.

My grandmother didn't care what ice cream did to her and was frequently found in the kitchen forcefully tugging on the lock. Regardless of where she was in the house, she had an uncanny sense of anyone moving in the general direction of the refrigerator. I never realized how often I randomly opened it myself until I had to enter a series of numbers each time for access.

Being deliberate about what I wanted, and quick and quiet in removing the lock, became an art form. Rotating the dial right, left, then right again, I'd think I was in the home stretch until my ears picked up the sound of Ma stomping down the hall. "Ughh," I'd groan as my fingers fidgeted nervously to get the shackle out and grab my food before she ambushed me.

My grandmother was stocky, but she could move. I had about a second to retrieve an item and replace the lock before she turned the corner into the kitchen and was bearing down on top of me, begging for ice cream. At the time, Ma was a little over five feet tall but physically robust and strong as an ox. As her disease progressed and she became more aggressive, the begging for ice cream advanced into a full-fledged wrestling match whenever that lock came off.

※ ※ ※

Ma grew up in a large family whose pastimes included playing games, mastering musical instruments, and singing. I never thought she could carry a tune, but it was obvious she didn't share this opinion. It was quite embarrassing as a kid if you landed next to her in church, where she belted out songs with the lung force of Whitney Houston. Hymns are often learned in childhood, and, apparently, hers were hardwired. Even with Alzheimer's, standing next to Mom, Dad, and me at Mass, she would proudly drown out all the pews around us with her "Our Fathers" or "Ave Marias." I didn't wince then, but I often caught my dad trying to suppress a laugh!

Card games were another serious business for Ma, and she had no patience for idle chat or delays making a move. She had an annoying habit of drumming her fingernails on the tabletop if someone was taking too long to decide. Then in their haste they would make a dumb move, and she would roar with laughter. She was a formidable competitor.

After her diagnosis, Ma never forgot her love for cards, but over time she forgot most of the rules. Often, she would line up several rows of cards horizontally as if to play solitaire. Flipping the cards from the remaining deck, she would chaotically place them all over the table—her confused state of mind playing out right before us.

Ma was still laughing at that point and occasionally winking at me when my mom got upset with her, which I found to be hysterical. She was half-adult, half-kid and fluctuated between the two. As seriously as my mom took this disease, it was hard not to laugh at some of the crazy things that half-kid did—and spoke! Erma was right, there is a fine line between comedy and tragedy, and we were all walking that tightrope, balancing the sadness of losing the Ma we knew with the lightness her new behavior often brought.

Chapter Six

A (Not So) Novel Disease

Science, my lad, has been built upon many errors; but they are errors which it was good to fall into, for they led to the truth.
Jules Verne

At first, Mom didn't understand the reason behind my grandmother's unusual behaviors, and her doctor wasn't much further ahead on education or information. Alzheimer's disease was a developing label in the early eighties that came with severely limited instructions and information.

The first case of Alzheimer's dates to 1906. It was named after Alois Alzheimer, a German psychiatrist and neuroanatomist who followed the progression of his patient, Auguste Deter, from hospital admission to her death five years later. This fifty-year-old woman was originally admitted with paranoia, aggression, and increasing sleep and memory disorders. While doing her autopsy, Alzheimer found her brain had shrunk. Under the microscope he observed abnormalities of her brain tissues, which he labeled as "distinctive plaque" and "neurofibrillary tangles."[14]

Unfortunately, medical politics of the day silenced his discoveries, and he died long before these findings would become the most plausible and researched culprit behind the disease. During that seventy-plus-year pause, research moved at a snail's pace, and a loved one displaying symptoms of confusion and memory loss after age sixty-five was considered to be going senile—a natural, intrinsic component of the aging process.

The Alzheimer's Association was formed in 1980 through the collaboration of Jerome H. Stone, members of family support groups, and the National Institute on Aging. Support for Alzheimer's research then began to grow in the private and public sectors. President Ronald Reagan used his platform in 1983 to bring the disease into the national spotlight by announcing the first official Alzheimer's Awareness Week. In 1984, a pathologist from the University of California at San Diego, George Glenner, and his colleague, Caine Wong, isolated the distinctive plaque and neurofibrillary tangles, first discovered by Dr. Alzheimer.[15] This gave birth to new labeling as beta-amyloid plaque and Tau, the harmful protein tangles formed inside of brain cells.

As Alzheimer's progressed in my grandmother, her care became overwhelming. Ma needed constant eyes on her, and Mom was still working. Mom tried to manage her schedule around whoever might be home to look after Ma, but Dad also worked, and my brother and I were commuting back and forth to college. The endless wandering, paranoia, and sleepless nights were increasing, setting everyone on edge.

Mom had stared down many adversities in life, and although this disease had gained more prominent recognition since Dr. Alzheimer first discovered the brain abnormalities of his deceased young patient, the new label of Alzheimer's brought no solutions, modest information, and even less support. Mom couldn't fight something she knew so little about. This mysterious force was taking over Ma's mind, slowly chiseling away at her and simultaneously eroding Mom's energy and resources. Alzheimer's was fighting on two fronts, and Mom's good intentions to keep Ma at home began to vaporize.

Broken by these harsh realities, my mom and her sister, Mary Jane, reluctantly set out to find other living arrangements. The places they visited ranged from smaller homes that cared for up to a dozen residents to larger, full-scale nursing facilities. I accompanied them on many of the tours, and all these places repulsed me; I couldn't imagine leaving my grandmother in any of them. Nothing met with Mom or her sister's approval either, but they were out of options. Wanting my grandmother close enough to visit every day after work, location became a priority.

Soon, a nursing home was found not far from my parents' and aunt's homes. The paperwork was signed, and Ma's fate was sealed, launching a horrific journey that would haunt our family for decades. The dubious day when Ma would leave our little cocoon, exposing the true horrors of Alzheimer's in the early eighties, loomed large on the horizon. There, our sweet Ma would slip into a rabbit hole so surreal and dark that she would never be found again.

Chapter Seven

The Nightmare Begins

I'd realized there were scarier things in the world than the monsters that lived in my nightmares.
Krystal Sutherland

Smell is one of the senses that cues us back to an event, and my grandmother's first nursing home was the kind of place you smell before you even walk in. As the glass doors slid open, the sweet and sickening stench of Lysol-masked urine greeted me. Past the reception desk was a common area that held an arrangement of tired and unmatched couches and chairs situated around a small TV. Residents there were either sleeping or staring blankly, but no one was really watching the program. Continuing down the corridor with its harsh fluorescent lighting, occupied wheelchairs lined both sides. The individuals in them held various positions from sitting up to slouching over to partially sliding through their restraints.

Moving closer to my grandmother's room, my ears picked up the forlorn cries of bedridden residents. Some were beckoning help while others just moaned. I tried not to peer in as I passed their rooms, but curiosity always got the better of me. I could never decide if they were in pain or just crying out for human companionship; either was heartbreaking. Moving through the lines of wheelchairs, I came across sweet residents who reached out their arms, and it was hard to ignore them. But if you held their hands, they refused to let go as they looked up at you with pleading eyes. That was devastating—and awkward—because pulling away seemed so heartless, leaving me to wonder how often, if ever, they received visitors.

Balancing out the pleasant folks were the angry ones who barked at me for simply looking at them or walking too close to their chair, causing me to quicken my pace. I really wanted to see my grandmother, but not there. Everyone was either sad or angry. They were each somebody who belonged to someone, somewhere, and they certainly didn't belong in that rathole of a place.

That said, I fully understand nursing homes are a safety net for many who have no other options, and moving was a necessary reality for Ma. Some facilities have come a long way over the past few decades, but the lifeless aura surrounding my grandmother's first nursing home overshadowed anything deemed beneficial—at least from my perspective.

The Nightmare Begins

There might have been splashes of color on the walls, but all I remember was gray: that overcast, dreary gloom that swallows you up on a lifeless winter's day. That's how I felt, engulfed in a cloud of despair and hopelessness. To me the place was nothing more than a waiting room for the dying, and the smell of death permeated my nostrils. My grandmother's last days and nights were going to be there, and, in my opinion, it was a horrendous place to live and to die. But this was a snapshot of the typical nursing home in the early eighties.

This was the literal dawn of Alzheimer's, when senility evolved from a normal aging process to a serious medical condition. Funding increased and researchers raced to understand the reason behind all of the strange behaviors in these confused individuals. Like any novel discovery, the data was developing, and information was scarce and confusing. My grandmother was part of that first generation whose only treatment consisted of a few older drugs, not created to treat dementia, that sent them into a stupor. Ma walked into that nursing home, but she never walked out and not because she died there.

This nursing home's drug of choice was Haldol, and it was given to control her wandering. It was a blanket drug, intended for psychosis, that addressed the vast spectrum of Alzheimer's-related behaviors. At first, it caused Ma to shuffle her feet when she walked, turning her into a zombie straight out of *The Walking Dead*, minus the theatrical gore. Her soles never left the ground as she shifted slightly from side to side, slowly progressing down the hall.

She wasn't alone in her unusual gait because, unless a resident was wheelchair bound, they all danced the Haldol shuffle. It was agonizing to visit her in those early days, as profound sadness hung over her. She cried when we arrived, begging us, "Please take me home." She then pleaded as we left, "Please don't leave me here. Please, please take me with you."

Mom nudged me along during those painful visits as the gut-wrenching sight of my grandmother crying and imploring us to take her home stopped me dead in my tracks. I hated seeing her like that, but it was even harder to watch Mom wrestle her demons over leaving Ma there. She put up a tough front, but I saw the stress in her face, the deep worry lines across her forehead that never softened, and the dark bags under her eyes from lack of sleep. You would think she'd sleep better knowing Ma wasn't roaming our house or neighborhood at night, but she never came to terms with moving Ma out. It was a no-win situation for both of them. Although Mom's struggle with this predicament was palpable, she didn't talk much about it then. But later, after Ma passed, she often lamented about her actions, saying things like, "I never should have moved her from our home. Why didn't I just let her live out her life with us?"

The depth of challenges surrounding Alzheimer's at that time completely overwhelmed both the staff at the nursing home and the medical community at large. In 1987 the first drug trial was introduced with the goal to intentionally address the symptoms of Alzheimer's, such as depression, anxiety, delusions, and paranoia. In my grandmother's case, as the disease progressed, the only option to control her symptoms and unwanted behaviors was to up her meds. Unfortunately, more Haldol meant more brutal side effects, blurring the line between the damage from the drugs and the degenerative effects of the disease. Paracelsus, the sixteenth-century Swiss physician and alchemist was correct with his well-known assertion on toxicology when he said that the dose makes the poison. We didn't call Haldol a poison then, but, because of its careless use with Ma, I certainly would today.

When Ma began to shuffle her feet, tremble, and drool, the medical staff attributed the decline solely to Alzheimer's. When her confusion increased to the point where she couldn't verbalize her words, they blamed it on Alzheimer's. When she couldn't walk and landed in a wheelchair, that too was a result of the disease. Therefore, the treatment plan for Ma to control the unwanted behaviors—such as agitation, aggression, wandering, and sleep disturbances—was drugs. And when that proved ineffective, ironically, the treatment plan for the drug-induced symptoms was to increase the dosage. Mom fought valiantly every time this happened but was always given an ultimatum: increase the dose or move Ma out. Since Mom's choice of facilities was limited by location, there was nowhere else to go.

This led my grandmother, and many others, to a wobbling, slumberous state which left them too groggy to walk and too confused to talk. Haldol is used sparingly today with Alzheimer's, which leads me back to Paracelsus and dosing, but I believe Haldol was improperly prescribed to my grandmother at that time and most likely because prescribing it was all that the medical community knew to do. When the gates of Alzheimer's opened in the early eighties, and the tremendous flood of patients came staggering through, health professionals were as overwhelmed as their patients were confused. Their only answer was to medicate and sedate.

Ma remained in her first nursing home until the mid-eighties. It was a nightmare that none of us woke from. Her claim to fame was an uncanny similarity to the great Houdini, becoming gelatinous as she slowly slithered out of her restraints, ultimately ending in a puddle on the floor. Her quality of life dwindled, and she wasted away until she became a shadow of her former self, the spunky and strong-minded grandmother I once knew. Reduced to simply existing, she was no longer a problem for anyone. The nursing home successfully *managed* her.

Patient narcotized, check.

Chapter Eight

The Final Goodbye

1992

Goodbyes are only for those who love with their eye.
RUMI

The entire experience of moving Ma from our home and into a nursing facility imbedded a deep and lasting fear in Mom of Alzheimer's and nursing homes. Mom was entangled in a sweeping anxiety which impelled her to make me swear, whenever the subject of Ma came up, that I would never put her in a nursing home. In fact, she stated more times than I could count that she would never go into one. I absolutely believed her because I knew my mom well, and that unwavering will of hers was not easily subdued.

She'd had to stand helplessly by as my grandmother drifted further into the deep void of Alzheimer's, and she was determined not to have that be her experience if she slipped into dementia. Regardless of whether the disease's progress was hastened or hidden by medication, there was no quality of life as Ma traversed that path. She was too medicated to use whatever part of her brain may not have been damaged by the disease, and if she experienced any glimpses of cognizance, she was too groggy to communicate them. Physically, she moved too quickly from walking freely to shuffling her feet and then to a wheelchair. She walked into that facility talking, but it wasn't long before she was blabbering gibberish, and that gibberish slowly gave way to a blank stare. Mom desperately wanted to connect with Ma, to believe she existed somewhere beyond her stupor, but she lost her early in the disease and the years slipped away. By the time experimental medications became available to address the symptoms, Ma was already in late stage.

※※※

In the mid-eighties, another type of senior care facility opened on the west side of the city near my parents' home. This was a retirement village that promised independent living through skilled nursing care. A new and emerging concept in eldercare with its origins in Denmark, this model was created to meet the needs of the senior population who wanted to "age in place"—the term used to describe a facility where you can move from independent living to assisted living and then to nursing or a combination of memory care and nursing. If you have the financial resources to stay, you never have to leave. But buyer beware: even if is affordable, aging in place is used loosely today by many institutions that do not have a dedicated nursing unit, as I unfortunately discovered shortly before Mom's death.

When Mom got word that the nursing floor of this new community had a waiting list, she leapt at the opportunity to add Ma's name. Soon after, a bed became available. Unlike my grandmother's first place, the nursing level here was top notch. There were two entrances to access Ma, but we preferred the main entry through independent living.

This approach invited us through a stylish and tranquil reception area with plenty of natural light—a far cry from the first facility. Warm cream tones accented with browns covered the walls. Beautiful paintings and indirect lighting provided by lamps and wall sconces greeted us on the way to the elevators. Residents of independent living were reading in the library, playing games in the family room, or having a bite to eat in the dining room. The common areas were richly appointed with stylish but comfortable couches and chairs in arrangements that enticed residents to rest, read, or play a game of cards. The dining room tables were covered in white linens and held small vases of fresh flowers. They even had a happy hour where the residents gathered around the piano, listening to music and sipping cocktails. Life was evident everywhere.

Although Mom's destination, where she would find Ma, was up the elevator to the nursing floor, the journey was more enjoyable and maybe even mentally prophylactic, like applying bug-spray before venturing out for a wooded stroll at sundown.

The independent residents appeared vibrant and seemed to enjoy their lives. Mom was quick to make friends with several of them while also connecting with others who were old friends of my grandmother before she'd developed Alzheimer's.

Mom didn't know a stranger. As an only daughter, I was her sidekick, which meant spending lots of time with her. No matter where we went, I listened to her converse with just about everyone we came across. She was an extrovert, and I wasn't, so it was often irritating as she rambled on about what I thought was nothing important. Listening to her talk with residents before visiting Ma was a different type of encounter. I sensed her need to connect and saw how it somehow lessened her stress, so I was happy to oblige. Occasionally, we came across Marge and Henri, a couple living in the independent wing who were old friends of Ma and my grandpa and whom Mom knew well. After they inquired about Ma, they often launched into a story about the good old days—the late-night card parties, the long phone calls between my grandmother and Marge. Mom would break out in a big smile as she recalled my grandmother's love for the telephone, especially after Grandpa died. "She could talk your ear off," Mom would always add, "and she never knew when to hang up!" That statement always brought a giggle to me as that signature habit was clearly passed on to my mom.

Mom looked forward to these interactions, often sitting down with anyone who inquired about my grandmother. This was her platform, and she had a captive audience with Alzheimer's so young in its narrative. The seniors wanted to know everything they could about this disease and Mom's experience with it, although the account probably unnerved some.

What struck me most was Mom's desire for others to remember the Mary Lambert (Ma) she knew and loved. It was blatantly obvious that Mom couldn't let go of that strong woman and mother figure, and probing the possibility that she still existed beyond the disorder helped her hold on to that persona. She wanted to believe that Ma was in there somewhere, and she never stopped trying to connect with her. However, there was very little, if any, acceptance of that mindset then. Recognition of Alzheimer's was in its infancy, and by all outward appearances the patient simply disappeared.

Mom was faithfully devoted to my grandmother and spoke in a manner that respected her maternal position, even at the end when she was bedridden and staring vacantly into space. "Mother" was the term used when addressing her, and Mom always acted as if she completely understood everything said—even if it was gibberish. She was quick to reproach us if we talked around Ma and not to her. Until the end, she held on to the hope that Ma heard her.

My grandmother's last years were unremarkable. She spent her days in a wheelchair being pushed from her bedroom to the common area, and then back at the end of the day, day after day. My lasting image of Ma is in this late stage. Strapped to a chair, she is leaning slightly forward with her arms bent at the elbow and crossed in front of her chest, as if in a hug. Sparse, thin strands of white hair are tucked behind her ears, and her lap is covered in a blanket. Those once brilliant blue eyes that continued through the succeeding generations had long since dimmed from the effects of Alzheimer's and medication; they were glassy and distant, leading me to wonder if Ma was still in there even if Mom was convinced she was.

But here's the evidence there was something going on deeper in Ma: her blank expressions, at times, transfigured into what appeared to be an awake mindfulness. I have pictures of my grandmother during her stay on that nursing floor, at her birthday and other holiday gatherings. Her children and their extended families with grandchildren and great-grandchildren surround her. Occasionally, the newest great-grandchild is placed on her lap and photos snapped. There is one that stands out in my mind. Ma is in her late eighties, and someone is holding my newborn son up to her. She is holding his gaze and looking intently into his eyes. I know that look because I have seen it in snapshots of myself and others as we first peered into our newborns' eyes. It's a collective expression of a visual engagement with a tiny soul so fresh from God: a primitive awareness of a love that has always existed.

If a picture paints a thousand words, then that photograph speaks volumes about the eyes of my grandmother's soul as she beheld my baby. Perhaps many cues fused together to fire up old neurons: the sight of an infant, the touch of his soft skin, and his intoxicatingly sweet baby scent. That incoming memory then opened a portal which sparked a familiar but ancient emotion of a deep and enduring love. A bygone, but still beholden to the ties of love that never sever. A connection forever captured in an image but escaping all of us at the time.

My grandmother was diagnosed with breast cancer in her last year, spending her final months bedridden. She lapsed into a coma two weeks before her death. In the moments before she died, Mom reported that Ma opened her eyes and attentively held Mom's gaze as she was sitting at the side of Ma's bed. Beholding each other in their concluding seconds as mother and daughter, tears softly flowed down Ma's cheeks before she exhaled her final breath.

Tears. Mom had waited a decade for a sign Ma existed inside the shell and it came in a cryptic form—tears represent the gamut of emotions from joy to grief. While it's clear Ma was yearning to express something important, that reason nagged at Mom for years. Trying to discern its significance, she often arrived at painful and negative conclusions.

Over time, I have come to a twofold opinion regarding those final tears. One probability is that in her closing moments, Ma experienced "terminal lucidity," which according to a "PubMed" article is "The unexpected return of mental clarity and memory shortly before death in patients suffering from severe psychiatric and neurologic disorders,…"[16] Experts are still investigating the reasons behind it, but it has been researched and reported in medical literature as far back as 250 years.[17] Personally, I also believe Ma's tears represented—and lamented—lost opportunities for communication and an overflowing appreciation for her family who stayed by her side but most especially for her beloved daughter who maintained a constant vigil during the lengthy journey.

Ma was gone. In her final act on the stage of this earthly drama she once again and for the last time disappeared into the night. This time Mom didn't call the police or alert the neighbors. Our faith placed my grandmother safely on the upward odyssey toward heaven. The core of my grandmother, the life Mom hoped still existed during her final grueling years on earth, was finally released by its captor—the prison of her body. Her last horse bet paid big as, forever light and free, she galloped away with the jackpot in sight.

We experienced deep joy at Ma's liberation from Alzheimer's. When a loved one stops suffering, a weight—perhaps unknown until it is no longer bearing down—suddenly lifts from the soul, even while mourning the person's physical presence. This should have freed Mom, but after a while it was obvious an indelible scar remained on her psyche. The post-traumatic stress, resulting from a decade of dealing with my grandmother's Alzheimer's, began to gnaw at her. My grandmother had passed, but the beast that first introduced itself as forgetfulness remained and continued to roar in the dark dwellings of Mom's brain.

Chapter Nine

The Beginning of the Bizarre

Circa 2000

*Nothing is so painful to the human mind
as a great and sudden change.*
Mary Wollstonecraft Shelley

"I found her garbage in my can! Gladys is putting *her* trash in *my* garbage can!" Mom complained vehemently into the phone about her longtime friend and next-door neighbor. Mom lived the greater part of her life next to the O'Brian family. Some fifty years earlier they were new neighbors with young, growing families. My parents built their home on Highfields Lane in the mid-fifties at the advent of both the Baby Boomers and suburban sprawl. The embodiment of post-war middle-class America, these homes were modest brick ranches and Cape Cods in planned neighborhoods that quickly became the focal point of family life.

Some fortunate families owned two cars but most owned one. Since the cars were used by the men during the day, the women relied heavily on each other for companionship and support. It was a village back then; the men went off to work in the mornings and the women spent their days cooking, cleaning, doing laundry, and tending to the kids. For all of us neighborhood kids growing up, everyone was our mom, and their watchful eyes were always upon us, ready to report any misconduct or even take matters into their own hands if need be.

In the event of an emergency, my siblings went to a neighbor's home while Mom escorted a child with a high fever to Dr. Fowler or one with a broken bone to the emergency room. If Mom ran short on flour or eggs while baking, one of us ran to the neighbor who had extra. When someone was sick, there was always a neighbor popping over to infer a diagnosis and possibly even share leftover antibiotics from one of their own kids.

I had colic as an infant, and, as the story was told, Mrs. Giordano, our neighbor to the right, brought over their rocking chair. She was always accompanied by Grandma Giordano who lived with the Giordano family. Grandma Giordano was always willing to share her many years of homespun wisdom—in this case, how to soothe an irritable and screaming infant.

My bedroom window bordered the back wall of our covered front porch, and many a summer's evening I drifted off to the sounds of Mom and a neighbor or two sitting on the gliders, chatting the night away. Such was the relationship between those strong and capable women who lived on Highfields Lane. They were extended family who walked alongside each other as they raised their families, commiserating hardships and celebrating joys.

Ultimately, the older kids grew up and moved out, leaving my brother Kevin and me at home when Ma moved in. The neighborhood was aging and began to take on the culture of an empty-nester community. My grandmother passed in 1990, and four years later my dad died of colon cancer while Mom was still in her sixties. Then, more than ever, the familiarity of the neighborhood and those enduring friendships became crucial to Mom and all of us kids.

Mom was quite comfortable living alone and thrived in that harmonious and protective environment. My brothers and I knew that the neighbors were watching out for Mom, as they had for my grandmother, as well as us kids growing up. It was reassuring to know that they were just steps away if Mom needed help.

So, of course, I was shocked when Mom started complaining about Gladys and the trash. The allegations were absurd, but I must admit the visual was comical as I pictured our eighty-year-old neighbor secretly planning her covert mission. Donned in all black, she waited patiently for the cover of darkness. Then, creeping past the trash cans behind her own house, she hopped the chain link fence that separated our yards. Once there—and with a heavy bag of trash in tow—she sprinted across Mom's driveway like a fox in hot pursuit of its prey. Breaking into the enclosed area under the second-story deck which housed Mom's green garbage cans, Gladys secretly deposited her trash then stole off into the night, a satisfied smile on her face.

While I could laugh at this imagined scenario with my siblings, I was irritated with Mom's crazy accusations and terrified she would confront our dear neighbors with this nonsense. I begged her to consider how outrageous she sounded, and how foolish she would look if she mentioned this to anyone. Of course, my brothers were hearing the same claims and calling her out, but the allegations didn't stop there. According to Mom, Gladys was also refusing to share her vine-ripe tomatoes from the garden and her famous fresh baked pies! In addition, Mom was quite certain that Gladys was no longer allowing her husband, Ronan, to talk with her.

Mom had a group of girlfriends from grade school that we considered family. They were all close, but one of her best friends was her cousin, Etty. I doubt many days went by when they didn't talk, or a week passed when they didn't see each other. However, during this time when Mom's pessimistic attitude was getting worse, even Etty wasn't safe from her negative onslaughts as Mom found opportunities to criticize her in some childish way.

Mom's list of offenders grew daily and the negativity, pettiness, and frequency of these troubling conversations increased. She was creating issues with individuals who had always been part of her inner circle, and once she latched on to an annoyance with someone, she couldn't let go. These types of behaviors slowly gained momentum until they started to define her, unfortunately, and then, to our horror, the more obvious signs of Alzheimer's started to appear. I was usually the recipient of Mom's rants, although my brothers got their fair share.

Typically, Mom's mornings began with walking her beloved ten-pound Bichon Frise, Abby, around the block. That dog went everywhere she travelled, whether she walked, drove, or flew. Mom would stop and chat with neighbors along the route, allowing Abby to complete her morning business, then they'd steadily make their way home. Once settled, Mom would prepare breakfast for the two of them in her bright yellow and blue kitchen. Pouring herself another cup of coffee, she'd sit at her little wooden table next to the large window that filtered in the morning sun. Eating hot oatmeal while sharing her banana with Abby, she'd begin her morning rounds of phone calls to family and friends.

I was living in Atlanta during that time and Mom's phone call was part of my morning ritual that I generally enjoyed. It was my daily dose of home that centered me, wherever I might be, anchoring me in the world I grew up in with ties to it that run so deep. After me, she would call my brothers, her cousins, and friends—likely anyone she could get through to. Mom loved to chat, in person or on the phone, which rightly earned her the nickname, "Chatty Patty."

During our call, Mom would share a funny story, tell me about her plans for the day, and inquire about my boys. She always insisted that I turn on *Good Morning America* so we could watch it together. She had a small TV mounted under her kitchen cabinets and alleged no morning was complete without coffee and her favorite show. Outside of the news, there was always someone interesting on or they were cooking up some delicious recipe she wanted me to try. Paula Deen was one of her favorite chefs, and my slightly "altered version" of Paula's pot roast recipe originated at Mom's insistence one cold morning as we watched *GMA* together—over the phone—and over breakfast! This was our early version of a Zoom call!

She loved to laugh and had this little ritual that started with my brother Joe. He would call Mom and let out a ridiculously silly laugh that got Mom laughing, and soon, they would both be laughing about nothing. She continued this with me and many others because she heard somewhere (probably on *Good Morning America*) that laughter was good for the soul.

I looked forward to Mom's morning calls, but, after a while, those pleasant, funny, and energizing conversations slowly transformed into disturbing, sad, and exhausting exchanges. She would complain about a situation, like the garbage, and become trapped in a dead-end of obsessive thoughts, judgments, and opinions. Her narrative circled a roundabout she was unable to exit. Meanwhile, I was stuck in the passenger seat. Her overall attitude and outlook on life became increasingly negative, and she began to show signs of paranoia.

That was when I began to dread her morning calls. I would see her number come up on caller ID and, for the first time in my life, hesitate to answer. My shoulders slumped as I let out a sigh, debating with myself as those rings piled up. What was worse: listening to her tirade or dealing with the guilt of not taking her call? I was raised Catholic, so guilt usually won out and I quickly picked up the phone before it went into voicemail.

As valuable as my grandmother's journey with Alzheimer's was, her early signs of the disease were different from Mom's (especially Mom's mounting attacks on some of her closest tribe), so we were thrown off track. Mom had always seen life in black and white, was staunchly loyal, and not afraid to express her opinion. She could be obstinate and quarrelsome at times, but up until this point always dealt in a reality that was within the realm of normal.

This was different. I knew the people and was familiar with the situations she was complaining about, and I recognized her version was distorted. Still, I never considered Alzheimer's. I instead attributed her negativity to the usual suspects: having too much time on her hands and possibly becoming bitter about being alone. Perhaps it was the latter part of dealing with grief over losing my father or just the normal aging process. I believed this because I had come across quite a few angry and unhappy senior citizens—not suffering from dementia—during my grandmother's tenure in nursing homes.

It's easy to miss these early behaviors until they begin to pile up and especially when not living with that person. Mom had little oversight as she tended to her days. My brothers and their families lived close by and were frequently involved with her, but she managed her life and made her own decisions. Outside of the increasing negativity though, she remained competent in maintaining her home, paying her bills, volunteering at the hospital, and walking daily. She always ate well, didn't miss a family event, and travelled extensively. After my dad passed, she spent a good part of the winters with my family in Georgia.

If she hadn't kept up in these other areas, perhaps we would have dug a little deeper. Those early signs are so elusive, and I know from someone close to me who has since been diagnosed that uncharacteristic behaviors in early dementia vary widely from person to person. Today, my grandmother's forgetfulness, confusion, and misplacement of items would easily signal a possible early dementia, but Mom's initial signs were more social in nature. Her growing negativity and mistrust of others was more annoying than concerning and so frustrating that I became more focused on trying to change her mindset than investigating why her behavior might be changing in the first place. Also, given what happened with Ma, I didn't want to believe that history could be repeating itself.

I can't pinpoint a date, but Mom's personality changes began several years before she was officially diagnosed, and, unbeknownst to us, these infuriating behaviors marked the beginning stages of a prolonged battle in her brain. This one-sided war with an unseen foe crept in unannounced, disguising its presence for many years. The enemy worked quietly behind the scenes, building an arsenal with weapons of destruction from within Mom's own body (anything that causes heart disease and reduced blood flow to the brain, such as high blood pressure, high cholesterol, diabetes), secretly seizing cerebral territory, and eventually obliterating everything in its path. While Mom was busy living her life, this clandestine operation to annihilate her brain cells was well underway and all within the confines of an otherwise beautiful existence.

Alzheimer's had a massive head start in Mom well before her bizarre behavior appeared. Complaining about, accusing, and distrusting her neighbors, friends, and relatives was a well-disguised symptom of a disease that conceals itself early-on while ravaging its victim's mental capacity. While researchers don't yet know its exact causes, they do know early signs can begin with subtle personality changes, well before the more obvious memory symptoms appear. Though my brothers and I didn't suspect dementia, Mom's crazy behavior with some of those closest to her caused a great deal of anxiety and unrest in her and those around her. Unable to recognize those early personality changes as signs of Alzheimer's—or any type of disease—I held Mom accountable for her actions and tried to reason with her whenever she went off on a tangent.

※ ※ ※

"Etty's husband is sick, and she is taking him to the VA hospital, instead of getting him proper care. She's just selfish and worried about saving money."

"Mom!!!" I shot back into the phone, not able to suppress my disappointment. You're talking about Etty, your lifelong best friend." The phone would go silent, and then I'd continue, thinking I was getting through to her. "VA care is good, and some of the best doctors train in their system. It's veterans caring for veterans," my voice much softer now.

"Well," she responded, "she only thinks about herself and doesn't care about him . . ."

This was not the Mom I knew, but it was the version of her I found myself encountering with increasing frequency. Mom was feisty, and had no issue voicing her sentiments about individuals she struggled with, but this behavior was out of character when it came to those she cared about the most. Unfortunately, her negative and fault-finding demeanor began to define her in the years before the more classic signs of Alzheimer's appeared. I'd fight her during these phone conversations—just as she'd bridled against Ma's nonsense—and try to show her a different angle or distract her altogether. But she'd only dig in deeper and defend her position. These conflicts were exasperating for everyone, but, looking back, no one suffered more than Mom as her relationships with those closest to her became a source of stress for her.

CHAPTER TEN

What I Wish I Knew Then (The Latest Data on Alzheimer's)

If we knew what we were doing, it would not be called research, would it?
ALBERT EINSTEIN

Today, evidence is clear that clinical changes in the brain are taking place decades before the actual diagnosis of Alzheimer's. Rudolph Tanzi, Director of Genetics and Aging Research at Massachusetts General Hospital, cited a study presented by an Australian team of researchers that tracked amyloid in the brains of individuals both affected and unaffected by Alzheimer's.

"What came out of that study was that amyloid accumulates in the brain 15 years before symptoms. So in these trials, you're treating full-blown Alzheimer's patients for amyloid, but amyloid had already accumulated, started the disease, and done its job. It's kind of like if you have a patient who has congestive heart failure or heart attack and they go to a cardiologist who says, "Here, just take this drug that will lower your cholesterol." It's too late. You had to have done that fifteen years before."[18]

The plaque Dr. Tanzi refers to is detected by means of a PET scan that "lights up" the amyloid plaques present in the brain of Alzheimer's individuals. This is a nuclear imaging procedure that releases a radioactive substance, called a tracer, into the blood by means of an IV. Before this imaging was available, the only way to accurately diagnose Alzheimer's was through an autopsy of the brain after death. Today, in addition to the PET scan that can diagnose the disease while the patient is living, there are ways to test for the presence of elevated amyloid levels in the blood *before* symptoms present themselves. An article from the National Institute on Aging,[19] states that amyloid in the brain can be tracked in several ways: through a blood test (which is the most non-invasive), a PET scan of the brain, and in the cerebrospinal fluid through a spinal tap. They go on to explain the benefits of this testing for people experiencing memory problems, and those diagnosed with mild cognitive impairment (MCI): it helps health care providers determine whether Alzheimer's is the potential cause, and also helps doctors respond with drugs that target amyloid. For people without any signs of dementia, and who may have a family history of the disease, the presence of amyloid plaque on the brain may help researchers enroll them in clinical trials for treatment to prevent or delay the onset of cognitive symptoms.

There are many terms used when talking about Alzheimer's and amyloid: amyloid theory, amyloid protein, amyloid plaque, amyloid-beta, and beta-amyloid plaque. All of which can be confusing. Amyloid is a protein normally produced by the body. In the brain, this protein naturally breaks down to form beta-amyloid fragments.

In a healthy brain, amyloid protein fragments are further broken down and removed, but not in the case of Alzheimer's. There are many forms of beta-amyloid, but beta-amyloid 42 is particularly harmful. When excess amounts of this protein cluster together, beta-amyloid plaque forms between the nerve cells, interrupting the communication, thus killing the brain cells. That's my simple interpretation, but the National Institute of Health (NIH) provides a thorough explanation of the process on their website.[20]

Adding to the complexity, there are also two types of the amyloid protein: soluble and insoluble. Soluble dissolves in water and insoluble becomes the sticky plaque that causes cell death. Many of us have both types in our brain, but not everyone with both the soluble and insoluble develops the disease. "The paradox is that so many of us accrue plaques in our brains as we age, and yet so few of us with plaques go on to develop dementia," said Alberto Espay, MD, a professor at the University of Cincinnati College of Medicine. Espay, together with Andrea Sturchio, MD, worked in collaboration with the Karolinska Institute in Sweden to publish their research findings. Espay goes on to explain that "Individuals already accumulating plaques in their brains who are able to generate high levels of soluble amyloid-beta have a lower risk of evolving into dementia over a three-year span.[21]

Beta-amyloid plaque, though originally discovered by Dr. Alzheimer in 1906, was not officially named until 1984. Since then, the financial backing for Alzheimer's research and development, heavily funded by pharmaceutical companies, has been directed exclusively toward this plaque. Scientists have brought forward other possible culprits of the disease but without success because the bullseye has remained on amyloid.

Thirty years later, and without a cure, scientists are at last considering other possibilities. In "What Causes Alzheimer's? Scientists Are Rethinking the Answer," researchers are looking beyond the amyloid theory as the primary offender: "Amyloid is more the smoke, not the fire . . . which continues to rage inside the neurons."[22] Researchers are also looking at Tau, a protein that stabilizes the interior skeleton of brain cells. When this protein stops doing its job, it attaches to other proteins causing Tau chains, or tangles inside the neurons, which also leads to neurodegeneration. "Alzheimer's is a disease of both amyloid plaques and tau tangles," says Brian Kraemer, PhD, a professor of medicine in the Division of Gerontology and Geriatric Medicine at the UW School of Medicine. "I think we must address both pathologies to see a therapeutic benefit for patients in terms of improved cognition.[23]

Dr Dale Bredesen, a globally recognized researcher and expert in the field of neurogenic diseases, including Alzheimer's, combines the traditional modes of medicine and research with a holistic approach. He believes Alzheimer's is not only preventable but also reversable and cites both anecdotal evidence and clinical trials to back up his views. His theories challenge the conventional medical wisdom of the day but also have shown remarkable results in their clinical trials.[24]

In a nutshell, Bredesen believes Alzheimer's, like many disease processes, is the result of multiple-system disruptions in the body likely beginning decades before symptoms appear. He identifies thirty-six of these disruptions which include inflammation, mold exposure, and diabetes. These are unique to everyone and should be addressed as part of the broader view of the disease. Since pre-symptomatic detection is an important part of his prevention and reversal strategy, Bredesen's advice is for everyone over forty-five to get a cognoscopy, (a combination of blood work, cognitive testing, and possibly brain imaging). In addition to testing for genetic markers, and beta-amyloid, these tests reveal the thirty-six possible disorders that contribute to one's risk for dementia-related decline. His methods for treating Alzheimer's focus squarely on those disorders, which he claims, when resolved or brought under control, can prevent—or even reverse—the disease.

I've often been asked, considering my history, if I would get genetic testing or check for beta-amyloid plaque in my brain. Not that having an accumulation of the plaque would signify a future with the disease, as twenty-five percent of people with plaque in the brain never get it. So, being free of symptoms, would I test? I think proactive testing for Alzheimer's takes a lot of courage, especially in the absence of a proven cure, and I admire individuals who choose to get tested. Asymptomatic testing is also critical for researchers conducting clinical trials, but I believe the mindset and mental health of an individual must be heavily considered.

Mom had many fears about getting Alzheimer's, a pervasive anxiety that was mentally taxing for her, but, if she'd been certain it was her future, years before her diagnosis and without a proven cure, I am confident it would have overwhelmed her life moving forward. I don't know if that type of cloud hanging over my head would be mentally detrimental or not, so I am still considering Dr. Bredesen's medically integrative methodology to testing.

In the meantime, implementing as many approaches as possible for improving my brain health is a daily practice (and sometimes a struggle). I start with some form of aerobic exercise (usually hiking with my dog and husband) followed by spiritual reading, meditation, yoga on some days, and trying to follow an anti-inflammatory diet, which is difficult when you have a sweet tooth![25] On the cerebral side of things, I am a voracious reader, love to write, research recipes, cook, entertain, garden, and spend time with those I love.

Sleep is also an extremely important part of the equation for brain, and overall health; it's when our bodies heal, and flush out toxins, especially in the brain.[26] I don't always sleep that well, but I attempt to do all I can to improve on that. I also try to be grateful for everyone, and everything, even challenging situations, for I know that's where I grow and evolve the most.

Last but not least, I am a firm believer in the power of letting go of what I can't control, which is almost everything! Both of those mindsets (when attained) help maintain my equanimity.

We learn from previous experiences, and I have benefited in ways too numerous to count from Mom's life and our journey with Alzheimer's. Mom ate healthily and was always on the go, but she didn't do well with quiet, reflective time or any down time, really. She had one mode, and it was MOVE. She often let trivial things get to her and didn't let them go too easily. Chronic stress, even on a negligeable level, has detrimental health effects on our body and psyche. Sleep wasn't an important consideration for her either; she often joked she'd sleep when she was dead!

I didn't know then what I know now, but, like most others, I did the best with the information I had at hand when caring for Mom. Realizing that, even though Mom suffered horribly in the earliest stages of this disease, brings peace. Unfortunately, Mom never found that, during or after her journey with Ma.

Research and clinical trials probe into the unknown hopefully to stumble upon a known—a discovery that will upend suffering—and make life more manageable or even better because of their findings. But, even without a cure, new information continues to improve the quality of life for everyone in this battle. One day, a crack will occur that allows the light to shine through the darkness we know as Alzheimer's. Until then, funding is the necessary fuel that keeps the pursuit moving forward.

Chapter Eleven

The Bizarre Has a Name

2003

*My eyes hadn't been looking. But now . . .
my mind could see without my eyes interfering.*
Leonard Seet

I love this quote. I don't know the author's intended meaning, but to me it's a truth about our overall psyche, which includes our ego's vested interest in maintaining stability. We see what we want to see, and when we don't see the obvious, it's often because we don't want to make real the unpleasant realities that change our world.

I didn't want to see my mom mentally failing, so I didn't look for signs, or, if I saw unusual behaviors in her, I made excuses for them. Mom was eighty-three years old and living independently in her home when my brother Tim finally became suspicious as he observed late notices on her kitchen table. Snooping around, he found stacks of opened mail lying in random places. There were piles on the kitchen counter by the phone, others on a desk in her back bedroom, and still more on the fireplace next to the mailbox that fed directly into her home. He even found bills in her car that she probably intended to pay directly, like Dillard's department store.

Luckily, she kept a substantial amount of money in her checking account because her checkbook was not balanced. She became careless about recording checks, which was unusual for Mom or anyone who grew up in the Great Depression era. Typically, she watched every penny spent, knowing exactly what monies came in and what went out.

Shortly after her checkbook fiasco, she began misplacing things, and if this bothered her, she certainly didn't show it. In fact, if we found her wallet in the refrigerator, the dog's chain in the laundry basket (which was always hung on a hook by the basement door), or her keys in the freezer, she would joke about it. I laughed with her about these things as Mom could be easily distracted.

This would have been more concerning if I hadn't known her so well and been accustomed to her thoughts racing ahead of her current activity. She wasn't always in the moment, which is certainly common for people under pressure or with a lot of responsibilities—continuously thinking ahead to the next box to check as they haphazardly drop their keys or glasses in some random place.

But this wasn't Mom's status, as the busy and chaotic days of raising kids and caregiving for Dad and Ma were behind her. Old mental habits die hard though, and our thoughts become runaway trains if we don't rein them in and *train* them to stay on task. It was easier to believe this was the case with Mom because, if it wasn't, then she was in trouble and her blithe attitude around misplacing things may have been denial. A fair denial, due to her past experiences with Alzheimer's, and one in which I rode the wake.

There is another disorder occurring in early Alzheimer's that looks a lot like denial. According to the Cleveland Clinic, "Anosognosia is a condition where your brain can't recognize one or more other health conditions you have. This condition isn't dangerous on its own, but people with it are much more likely to avoid or resist treatment for their other health conditions."[27] Presently, I am aware that I can't remember everything I need from the grocery store, so I make out a list. I am very aware that I am sweaty and smelly after exercise, so I take a shower. I don't want to forget appointments, birthdays, and other important dates, so I mark them on my online calendar, usually attaching multiple timed alarms starting a few days out from the event. I was concerned when my elderly neighbor, Sophia, began leaving Post-it notes, reminders to lock the doors and set the house alarm at night. I know now that Sophia's awareness of her forgetfulness, and the measures she took to compensate were the correct response to her age-appropriate memory loss.

Anosognosia is a matter of awareness, and the lack of awareness signifies a problem that affects more than half of all Alzheimer's patients early and to differing degrees. So, what looks like denial may be an organic manifestation of the disease. While anosognosia was a possibility with Mom, she often had an awareness of her forgetfulness. Frequently, she would stop mid-conversation as she struggled to find the right word then sail smoothly into another topic as if the original conversation didn't exist. Forgetting a name or word occasionally happens to all of us with healthy brains, although we usually recall the name of the person or the thing we were struggling to remember even if it pops into our consciousness later.

When Mom couldn't remember something directly asked of her, she often responded with a comment that deflected. For example, when I would ask her what she had for breakfast that morning, she would hesitate then respond with a statement like, "Oh, I rarely eat breakfast." But Mom didn't miss a breakfast in her entire life as she was part of a culture that believed it was the most important meal of the day. Mom was digressing, straying away from acknowledging she was struggling to remember. Although this must have terrified her, adversities throughout her life made her strong, and she took pride in that strength. She was convinced she could overcome anything with her unyielding will, and I am sure a failing mind was no different.

Like dominos falling into each other, the more traditional signs of dementia began to appear and pile up, sending Mom's symptom gauge into the red zone. The new status was GAME

ON, so we set up an appointment with Mom's primary care physician to investigate. Knowing it would be a struggle to get her there for reasons of memory loss, we convinced her she needed a yearly physical, and she agreed to go. It didn't hurt that Mom really liked her attentive, young doctor, and my brothers notified him of her symptoms ahead of the appointment.

Based on my brothers' reports, cognitive testing performed in the doctor's office, imaging of her brain, and bloodwork to rule out any other underlying diseases, Mom was diagnosed with mild cognitive impairment (MCI). According to the NIH, "Some older adults have more memory or thinking problems than other adults their age. . . . There is no single cause of MCI. The risk of developing MCI increases as someone gets older. Conditions such as diabetes, depression, and stroke may increase a person's risk for MCI."[28] This diagnosis doesn't always signal impending Alzheimer's, and some folks never go beyond it. But more people with MCI do go on to get Alzheimer's than those without. I was hopeful Mom was one of the lucky ones who wouldn't progress much further.

I was wary of slapping a label on Mom's forgetfulness as anything other than MCI, at least at the time. I didn't want anyone jumping the gun by assuming she was heading toward Alzheimer's because that's when drastic measures are taken. Sometimes changes are hard to roll back, like selling homes and cars, so I wanted to go slow. With a little oversight, she could live independently unless conditions changed and then we could, if necessary, deal with those changes.

At the time, and most likely because of her past experiences with Ma, Mom wasn't buying her diagnosis. She refused to talk about recent memory issues and didn't accept her doctor's conclusion—more denial. She called it nonsense, and her once-favorite young doctor would soon be added to the growing list of individuals conspiring against her. In her mounting paranoia, she believed her family was colluding with him to take away her independence.

"He's just like all the rest of you, trying to take away my car and put me into an old person's home," she would say.

"Mom," I would respond, "No one's trying to put you in an old person's home. We're all just concerned you're getting forgetful and need a little help. Your doctor's not making this stuff up; he ran tests, and the results don't lie." But there was no convincing her.

"Well," she quipped, "you're the crazy ones. There is nothing wrong with my memory, and I'm not having it."

She was living independently but dropping the ball on smaller details that easily go unnoticed when alone. Her refrigerator lacked the healthy options of food usually stocked, and the quantity of pills in her prescription bottles didn't match the number remaining according to the fill date. Some of her neighbors also voiced concerns that she was "somewhat erratically" driving up and down the street.

Soiled spots from her dog began appearing on her normally impeccable white carpeting, which meant Abby was not getting out on time. That led us to wonder if she was remembering to regularly feed her little friend. We didn't worry too much about Abby though because she was as headstrong as her owner, usually demanding food with loud continuous barking, earning her portions of Mom's food at every meal.

After Mom's MCI diagnosis, my niece and Mom's granddaughter, Brianne, a young adult at the time, moved into Mom's lower level to keep an unobtrusive eye on her. She provided Mom company in the evenings as they watched TV, and they took some meals together. This allowed a discreet supervision of Mom and her medications. Mom loved Brianne and certainly appreciated the company, but, while forgetful, she was keenly aware of the motivation behind Brianne's stay. "Being babysat," in Mom's words to me, was more than her pride could handle, and unfortunately that bandage came off.

Outside of keeping Mom home, the other solution was moving her to a full-scale retirement community that offered progressive levels of care. She could start off in independent living with a part-time aide or even a camera that watched her take morning and evening meds set out by a family or staff member. She would then be able to move toward increasing levels of care there as her disease progressed. My brothers explored that possibility and toured nearby senior living communities with Mom but to no avail. Mom was obstinate in her resolve to remain in her home, and alone. She was not going into any type of retirement community, which in her mind equated to a nursing home. Her only acceptable scenario was to live by herself without help or meddling from anyone, including family.

Mom's craziness had a name and that was important for her future, but she was in an early, transitory stage where she didn't need full-time care, only oversight in the specific areas where she struggled. Her inability to accept her diagnosis coupled with her strong desire for independence made it difficult to step in and make changes. It was a challenging time for the family, and we were somewhat divided on how to move forward. Given what we'd been through with Ma, my personal opinion was that we couldn't just rush in and make demands and decisions about Mom's life. Not yet.

Chapter Twelve

The Game Changer

2008

Not everything that is faced can be changed.
But nothing can be changed until it is faced.
James Baldwin

There are pivotal moments in life that change our direction. Sometimes, as with a health scare, they are thrust upon us and we immediately pursue a treatment or cure. Then, to keep that situation from ever happening again, we reevaluate our life, which often alters our way of living and thinking. Other times, those transformative events are discovered in hindsight and usually pinpoint back to a specific occurrence that set us on a different path.

Mom's moment came during a routine drive she'd executed successfully for decades. When it happened, the second shoe that was dangling in our family's Alzheimer's saga dropped. I heard it hit the ground but walked around that shoe for a while, observing it closely. Did it match Ma's? I wasn't sure but some of my siblings were convinced it did. Even so, I wanted indisputable proof because I knew that hasty extreme decisions would have far-reaching consequences for Mom, and she deserved that consideration. Was this situation confirmation that Mom was progressing beyond MCI?

Mom had stopped at a gas station and called my brother Joe, informing him she couldn't find her way to her cousin's. This wasn't her fault, she went on to say, because the street signs were changed and that confused her. That call in turn launched a series of others to my brothers and me. When I answered, Joe informed me Mom got lost driving. While initially alarmed then assured of her safety, I felt anger well up at my brother for delivering such a message.

Did he realize what he was implying? Joe was releasing the cap from a bottle that held all the horrors and sufferings of our grandmother's Alzheimer's—ghouls from the past just waiting to escape. I argued with him, not believing Mom really got lost driving, and told him he was making a mountain out of a molehill. I defended Mom because I was certain there was a reasonable explanation.

Perhaps the landscape changed and that had thrown her off. Maybe old buildings were torn down and trees wiped out, making way for a new neighborhood or strip mall, or any number of other things. I knew it was possible because I have encountered that scenario especially in a good economy with explosive new development. Driving a familiar route, I'd become distracted by my thoughts, talking on the phone, or selecting music. I'd come back to the present moment and suddenly find myself in a setting drastically different from the last time I was in it. The experience was surreal at first, and it would take me a second to get my bearings. Mom was older and her brain wouldn't process as fast. She panicked, that's all, and it happens to everyone. That's what I told my brother—and myself—and I was sure it was the case.

I tried so hard to keep Alzheimer's safely tucked away and hidden in the dark place where it belonged because there it couldn't touch Mom, or me, or my brothers. But Joe's call, even though at first I'd denied its implications, brought it painfully into the light. It was my moment of realization, but at the time it was blocked by my fears. The illumination of this emerging reality would be like gazing at an eclipse of the sun—staring directly was going to hurt—and I still needed blinders. Watching Mom go down this path was too overwhelming for me to consider, even as her new truth was taking form.

It might seem counterintuitive, but it takes a lot of energy to look the other way when faced with a grim diagnosis. I was clutching to life with Mom as I knew it by not acknowledging the signs that were snowballing. My blood boiled whenever anyone suggested Mom was moving toward Alzheimer's although I tried hard to suppress my rage. Being startled out of a deep sleep in the middle of the night because I dreamt something terrible had happened to Mom was a common occurrence. Then worrying that something actually had happened, until I was able to call her in the morning, was wreaking havoc on my nights and days. My body experienced a truth my head wouldn't admit: that's how denial works. It's an unpleasant reality wrapped up in a pretty bow, and, while it buys more time to maintain the facade, the smokescreen eventually dissipates, revealing the ugly truth. Mom's pretty bow was coming off.

As Joe disclosed the details of that ill-fated trip I closed my eyes, sucking in a deep breath. I could only imagine Mom's panic before summoning the courage to make that call. Disoriented, she became an amnesiac, unable to recognize her surroundings. Desperate to find some sign, a house or church or anything familiar to her, she turned left, then right, and then backtracked. I knew Mom put off that inevitable phone call for as long as she could because she had a strong aversion to admitting defeat, and an admission of that magnitude was certainly her last resort. Blaming the street signs for her disorientation was the act of a desperate woman too terrified to admit she was walking in the footsteps of the one before her. I understood that, but the fear of Mom hurting herself, or others, finally dispelled any lingering denial in me.

Today, because of smart technology, Mom could have easily pulled up an app on her phone and plugged in her cousin's address. Then, a friendly voice would have led her, step by step, safely to her destination. Google Maps or Waze would have enabled her to outrun that storm, but other storms, like planes lining up to enter the runway, were queued up and ready to fly. Mom was their destination.

We will never know how many risky situations Mom experienced before that day, but the thought of her harming herself or someone else while driving couldn't be ignored. The alarm was sounding, and I didn't have the code to make it stop. The family consensus declared she was teetering at the top of a very slippery slope and safety measures needed to be taken. The situation had changed, and my hesitation gave way to realization. It was time, and the difficult conversation with Mom was scheduled—another conversation no child ever wants to have with a parent.

Chapter Thirteen

The Conversation and the Fall

2008

There are choices we make, choices that are made for us, and things we ignore long enough until all choices have fallen away.
Neal Shusterman

Mom was running fast, glancing back at the dark clouds racing toward her—dark, spinning, ominous clouds releasing angry, white bolts of lightning—threatening to destroy life as she knew it. Sometimes, storms can be outrun. Warning sirens fill the air and the sound of thunder looms in the distance. The smell of danger permeates the air as large drops of rain begin to fall seconds before we reach shelter. Other times, despite valiant efforts, wrathful squalls surround and overtake us. Clouds open and torrents of rain crash down as lightning bolts strike even closer. Darting from tree to tree we're aware of their deceptive shelter, yet the facade of cover is the only thing we know. Mom couldn't find refuge; she was engulfed by the storm.

※ ※ ※

"Mare, Mom fell and broke her arm." My sister-in-law Cathy called to inform me that Mom had fallen on her front porch. Falls were not new to Mom as she had been losing her balance at times for no obvious reason since her seventies. She would go down hard and without warning. This time, unable to stop herself, she wound up flat on the ground.

It's an amazing yet scary phenomenon to observe someone fall like this. Mom was walking one moment then face-planted the next, and it happened in the blink of an eye. Growing clinical research strongly suggests that numerous falls and problems with balance, gait, and visual perception may surface in the pre-clinical phases of Alzheimer's—those years when Mom's personality began to change but before the more obvious signs of memory decline occurred.[29]

Cathy went on to explain what transpired before the fall. Mom was sitting on her front porch with a few of my brothers and probably thrilled they were spending time with her. Although recently diagnosed with MCI, she was certainly not aware of the family dialogues occurring around her. Consequently, she was not prepared for the life-changing conversation about to take place. My brother, Pat, a psychologist in Phoenix, flew in to facilitate the discussion that the family had all agreed on. He began to address her recent memory issues. These are difficult conversations to have with loved ones, especially when they don't know or won't admit they're having problems.

As one would expect, Mom's dander rose with the mention of a subject as sensitive as memory difficulties, but it hit its summit when they expressed their concerns around her driving. They continued the dialogue, trying to ease her anxiety by suggesting scenarios to keep her living independently at home. One was hiring a part-time aide who would visit daily. This person could take her shopping or wherever she wanted to go, help with light cleaning, and oversee meds. Supplementing this idea were senior day programs specifically designed for individuals with early dementia. These programs offered many stimulating activities for others at similar cognitive levels, allowing Mom to get out on weekdays. Of course, with so much family around, Mom would never be alone on weekends. They were good options but non-starters with Mom, whose mind closed at the mention of losing her beloved car.

Since driving was the major concern for our family at that moment, we'd gone back to her primary care doctor with the hope he could help us revoke her license. It's heartbreaking when these steps have to be taken, effectively treating the parent as a child. Legally though, her doctor could only recommend to her that she not drive based on her documented dementia. Because she wasn't buying that diagnosis, she didn't trust anything that came from him.

The state of Ohio doesn't mandate physicians report individuals who are cognitively impaired to the Department of Motor Vehicles (DMV), and as of this writing only about 13 percent of states require reporting although 50 percent encourage it.[30] Many doctors are uncomfortable disclosing this info to the DMV due to long-term patient relationships, which places the responsibility back on the family. Even if a state does mandate reporting, the DMV doesn't always completely revoke a driver's license, sometimes only suspending it and other times placing conditions on driving. It varies from state to state, but, typically, after a driver turns seventy they must renew their driver's license every three years, and the only requirement is a vision and written test. A road test will only be administered if a doctor, relative, or even a neighbor requests one on someone else's behalf.

Mom was outraged at the audacity of her sons' threatening to take her car away, and she began arguing. She was a born fighter who rarely lost an argument, and now her independence was on the line. Her radar was on full alert that sunny afternoon, sitting between her sons. She detected the enemy and it was in the form of her own brood. She began preparing a defense of her base because she knew a mutiny was ahead.

This was her front porch, her house of more than fifty years where she raised, clothed, and fed those very boys who were now making demands and decisions that were none of their business. She adamantly articulated that no one—especially her children—was going to tell her what to do or take away her car. She was completely capable of making her own decisions and caring for herself; besides, she didn't go that far, only to church, the store, and her sons' homes.

"I've never had an accident," she told my brothers, and repeated to me many times. "I don't need anyone driving me anywhere, much less living in my home, or coming in to help me. And I most certainly am *not* going to attend any kind of adult day care, no matter how you sugar-coat it. I just want everyone to leave me alone."

This looked like flat out defiance, and, initially, when she barked those remarks into the phone, I reacted in kind.

"Mom, we are just trying to help you, but your stubbornness, as usual, is getting in your own way."

However, the more she uttered those words, the more I heard her pain come through, and the more my stance softened—as did my awareness of her desperation. I could feel it, and it broke my heart. She was frantically trying to hold on to her independence, to the only life she knew and so dearly loved—that beautiful life that was slowly vanishing before her eyes.

Mom's reaction was reasonable for someone who doesn't remember the whys of a situation—why we wanted to take her keys away or why she couldn't live alone without help. But, beyond failing cognition, it's also a typical response when our senior loved ones feel their independence is being threatened. Nothing endangers autonomy quite like losing our wheels, leaving us at the mercy of others to get around. We come into life totally dependent on others but work hard to reverse that reliance, starting at an early age. I initially saw this attitude in my toddlers, some more than others, as they demanded that life run on their terms not mine. That need for independence increased as they got older until finally, at some point post-college, assuming all their own bills and chock full of responsibilities, they were at last delivered from dependency on Mom and Dad. No one wants to go backward.

We work our entire life to maintain that self-governing position, clinging to and preserving it, especially as we get older. Then comes the day when those very kids who couldn't wait to get out from under their parents' thumb, place them under theirs. That's when we really understand independence—when we're under threat to lose it. Mom was there.

Having had enough of their opinions and suggestions on how she should live her life, Mom abruptly rose from the chair on her front porch, an indication the conversation was over. She was visibly upset as she made her way to the front door, perhaps miscalculating a step or dizzy from the distressing conversation, and, before anyone was able to react, Mom was down. Not able to break her fall, she was once again prostrate on the ground, but this time with her arm caught under her body, twisted, and broken.

The fall led to a course of action similar to any injury that results in immobilization and rehabilitation. The break in Mom's humerus bone left her unable to use her dominant arm, to be alone, and to perform the most basic functions of daily life: dressing, bathing, cooking, and going to the bathroom by herself. The fall also left her unable to drive—and although this was an intended outcome, no one was happy about the painful way it transpired.

We employed part-time home health care aides who spent the day with her as she recovered, and my brothers and sisters-in-law took turns cooking and caring for Mom at night. But within a short time, she was flying the friendly skies to Atlanta, Georgia, where, unbeknownst to her, she would live out the rest of her days.

Mom didn't know it at the time and neither did we, but fate intentionally intervened that sunny afternoon on her porch. It commandeered the conversation and clearly conveyed what my brothers could not. Mom would never drive again.

CHAPTER FOURTEEN

HOME REDEFINED

Spring 2009

Very truly I tell you, when you were younger you dressed yourself and went where you wanted; but when you are old you will stretch out your hands and someone else will dress you and lead you to where you do not want to go.
(JOHN 21:18 NEW INTERNATIONAL VERSION)

Mom was trying to tell us something; her lips were moving, but her speech was slurred. She had just arrived at our home with Cathy after a short flight from Cincinnati. Much of our extended family was also coming to town for the weekend to celebrate two college graduations and a sendoff for our oldest son who was entering the military.

Mom was under the assumption she was coming to Atlanta for a party and then remaining for a short period while she rehabbed her broken arm. She was clearly in high spirits as she walked in our home. Making wide and sweeping gestures with her hands, she enthusiastically tried to communicate but was oddly not able to clearly articulate the words. I shot Cathy a questioning look, and she whispered in my ear that Mom's current state started sometime after touchdown in Atlanta.

We sat Mom on the sofa, trying to lower her unusually high energy level. She was always excited to travel, so this wasn't too much out of the ordinary, but that night she was in rare form. She gladly accepted hot tea, and as we gathered around her on the couch, she began to calm down. She wasn't experiencing numbness or weakness in her limbs, didn't seem off balance, and her vision was fine. After a brief period, she recovered and began speaking normally. Mom's symptoms came and left quickly. If she'd been alone, she may not have recognized or even remembered having trouble articulating her words. When we brought it up the next day, she denied it ever happened.

Mom's indecipherable babbling was most likely caused by a transient ischemic attack (TIA), also referred to as a mini- or warning stroke. According to the Mayo Clinic, a "TIA is a brief blockage of blood flow to part of the brain, spinal cord or the thin layer of tissue at the back of the eye known as the retina. This blockage may cause temporary stroke-like symptoms. But a TIA doesn't damage brain cells or cause permanent disability. This is how it differs from a regular stroke. A TIA is often an early warning sign that a person is at risk of stroke. About 1 in 3 people who has a TIA goes on to experience a stroke. The risk of stroke is especially high within 48 hours of a TIA."[31]

The symptoms from a TIA are mild, lasting only minutes, and in most cases the person is unaware of what is happening. Unlike a regular or ischemic stroke, the immediate impairment occurring with TIAs, such as slurred speech or trouble understanding speech, vision changes, problems with balance, numbness on one side of the body, or severe headache, is not usually permanent and typically resolves itself quickly. But the long-term effects can cause issues. "New findings from the University of Birmingham challenge the 'transient' nature of mini-strokes and provide insight into the long-term impact of an under-recognized condition. TIA patients in the study consulted their GPs [General Practitioners] more frequently than similarly aged patients for fatigue, cognitive impairment and anxiety or depression."[32]

Mom recovered rapidly, but a later MRI revealed that she had been having these TIAs for some time. Predictably, since she lived alone and denied having health issues, she never complained about experiencing unusual episodes. She was rarely ever sick, and, outside of multiple skin cancers, was physically very healthy. She certainly didn't voice concerns to her doctor. Because the symptoms disappear quickly, if Mom noticed any at all, she more than likely thought it was something else. Similar symptoms that mimic TIAs could result from a migraine, a seizure, or syncope, which is a rapid fall in blood pressure that causes dizziness or unconsciousness. Syncope is usually a cardiac issue and can be experienced in individuals on blood pressure meds who get up too quickly from a bending or sitting position. Mom's unexplained stumbling and falls may have been an indication of TIAs where she experienced unsteadiness before the fall, but she never said she was dizzy. She always blamed it on being clumsy, which she occasionally was, so we didn't make the connection.

In 2009, Mom was taking an aspirin every night, but today she most likely would have been put on anti-platelet, or blood thinning, medication to prevent further occurrences of TIAs or even an ischemic stroke. TIAs and ischemic strokes are most commonly associated with vascular and mixed dementia, the latter being a combination of Alzheimer's and vascular dementias, which is what I believe Mom had.

True to form, Mom was up early on the morning following her arrival in Atlanta with coffee in hand and party hat on! Any remnants of symptoms from the night before had vanished, and she was busy talking about the festivities ahead. She loved celebrations of any kind: weddings, baptisms, graduations, holidays, birthdays. She was always ready at the drop of a hat and planned for those occasions with trips to the mall. There, she would spend hours searching out the perfect gifts and outfits. Whenever I mentioned that we were planning something, and before I had a chance to extend an invite, Mom's swift response was always, "When should I be ready?" Assuming she was always included, she never waited to be asked.

Leaving Cincinnati and heading to Atlanta with Cathy for a long weekend of celebrations along with a little rehab on her arm was an easy sell. We were expecting many guests and had a full weekend of activities planned. Mom had her own suite on our home's main level that she and her pup occupied for parts of winter and various other durations since our move to Georgia. All the boys were home, and we had a house full of family and friends in and out all weekend. Mom was exactly where she flourished the most, right in the center of all the fun and commotion.

On the day following her arrival, I talked to her about staying with us until her arm healed and she completed physical therapy, which was another six months. I explained that we'd retrofitted her bathroom, making it easier for her to navigate while she recovered. I laid out all the fun adventures planned that summer and fall: trips to the mountains and beach, outdoor concerts, plays at the Fox Theatre, and outings to museums. I told her we would resume luncheons with my girlfriends and their moms, whom she always enjoyed seeing. Maybe the best enticement of all was shopping! With several beautiful malls within a twenty-minute drive of our home, there was lots of shopping for us to do.

I always lured Mom with plans she looked forward to. She thrived on hustle and bustle, always wanting to go, go, go, and I made sure to keep her busy whenever she came to town. This visit, however, was more challenging because, for the first time ever, Mom was anxious about being away from her home. I really had to elevate my pitch for this stay to sound attractive.

Although she never talked about the porch conversation with my brothers, it was clearly weighing heavily on her mind. She was suspicious about staying so long with me but agreed to the plans because she knew she couldn't care for herself without the use of her right arm. When she reluctantly consented, she was quick to add the stipulation that she intended to go home just as soon as her arm healed.

"I still have a life in Cincinnati, which I plan on resuming. That's where my house and car are, and when my arm is healed, I'll be fully able to take care of myself."

She was adamant about what she wanted, and that certainly didn't include spending the rest of her days with me. I understood where she was coming from. She wanted to live out her life in the place where she had spent her last fifty years. She sought everything that entailed: driving herself to the market, church, and walking Abby around her neighborhood while chatting with lifelong neighbors. She wanted to continue meeting with her grade school friends every Wednesday for breakfast and sit on her porch at night, watching the younger generation play in the cul-de-sac just like her own kids did. She couldn't understand why that was so hard for everyone to grasp—and that made her angry. Her paranoia, often directed at people close to her, made matters worse.

She wanted her life, not mine, and it made perfect sense because I hope for the very same thing. Much like the words of John 21:18, I want to dress myself, go where I want, and make my own decisions. Mom was fighting for her freedom, and because of that I needed to preoccupy her days with activities and her mind with prospects of enjoyable experiences. I didn't have the heart to tell her the truth because she never would have agreed to it. Our days together would have then become one long knock-down-drag-out battle of the wills. Dementia was damaging Mom's memory, but it didn't diminish her passion and her fight response was strong as ever.

There are different kinds of truths in life, and some hold a higher degree of importance than others. Telling Mom she'd never go home was a straightforward truth, but an overriding truth questioned her cognitive ability to weigh the pros and cons and arrive at a reasonable solution. The higher truth considered her mental health, as well as mine, and banked on another truth: the sad reality that Mom would eventually forget her home in Cincinnati and all the reasons she loved it so.

Our plans would keep Mom in Georgia for the remainder of her life, and sometime after her move to Atlanta, her life in Cincinnati was sold or given away—car and home—everything. Only her family and friends remained. She was never told. Meanwhile her mind was still flashing pictures and videos of her little yellow-brick house and sporty black sedan sitting in the garage—memories that were causing us both grief. I knew this was the right thing to do, and it was in Mom's best interest, yet it still felt like a betrayal. On one hand I struggled with Mom's right to consent about her care and other decisions, but on the other I knew she was quickly moving beyond her cognitive ability to be objective. Alzheimer's turned back the hands of time to a period, much like in childhood, where she could no longer discern her best interests.

Unfortunately, because there is no gold standard in determining competency in decision-making with this disease, the door remains open—often for years—to uncertainty and doubt. But herein lies the fringe benefit of a failing memory, one not offered by most other degenerative and life-ending diseases. This dubious advantage breaks through the ceiling of indecision because Alzheimer's follows a predictable path although with varying timelines. Maintaining this long-range view allows decisions to be made well in advance, giving early resolution to housing options, advance directives, trusts, financial and health care powers of attorney, and ultimately, end of life decisions.

With Mom on this foreseeable and inevitable path, my family could bank on her failing memory to erase, and thereby sever her attachment to, most of what she currently remembered. If I could mentally survive the interim, I knew at some point she wouldn't stress and fight about matters she sadly no longer recalled. This was either the most cowardly or compassionate way out, and I continually vacillated between these two perspectives, eventually coming to the realization that it was necessarily both. There is an old proverb, a universal truth that says time heals all wounds, and this especially applies to Alzheimer's. Time allows the cognitive loss to advance, taking with it the anxiety typically found in early to moderate forms of the disease. Starved of the anguish that comes from remembering and yearning for a past life, Mom would eventually become more peaceful.

Thanks to my grandmother, and that generation of souls who first staggered down the Alzheimer's path, we were able to prepare for what was likely to be Mom's future—even without a formal diagnosis of Alzheimer's, as that would come later. Those early pioneers blazed the trail when the forest was dark and dense with thickets and vines, leaving behind a path wide and clearly marked. Ma allowed us to stand on her shoulders and see Mom's and care for her in a fashion that was much more humane than what my grandmother ever experienced. She would have wanted that for her daughter, and, in some strange way, just knowing that gave Ma's horrendous journey a purpose.

Mom was home, not her definition of home nor a place of her choosing, but in a space that held her safe within a circle of love that would protect and embrace her until she transitioned to her eternal dwelling. There was a plan in place, a direction forward amidst a disease that works in reverse. This approach would take her by the hand as she staggered through a chapter she never wanted to read—nor did I. I only wanted to turn back the hands of time to that place where Mom was healthy, and, for one last time, hold tightly to what I would have to leave behind.

Chapter Fifteen

Could It Be This Easy?

Summer and Fall 2009

So, in a curious lurid calm which could not last and yet, it seemed, could not end, the days went by.
Iris Murdoch

Before Alzheimer's, Mom spent a good part of her winters with my family since our move from Cincinnati to Atlanta in the late nineties. She'd arrive shortly after New Year's with her beloved Abby in tow and stay until the frozen ground in Ohio thawed, usually in early spring. She easily integrated into our lives and really enjoyed being with the family. She loved the boys, and they adored her. I grew up with five brothers and had three sons, so trust me when I say I really enjoyed having another female in the house!

Mom was an early riser, up and out of her room at the crack of dawn no matter how late she stayed up. She either didn't require much sleep or lived her life tired, which was the more likely scenario as she pushed her way through fatigue to avoid missing anything. I frequently suggested she take a nap, particularly when we had a lot going on, and selfishly because I wanted one myself, but she always declined the offer. I jokingly referred to her as the Eveready Battery because she never seemed to run down.

Although we teased Mom about always being the last to bed and the first up, a lack of sleep is no laughing matter for many reasons, including its effects on and role in dementia. Numerous studies, including one by the NIH, demonstrate how lack of sleep leads to an increase of beta-amyloid accumulation in the brain.[33] There are individuals who genetically require less sleep. Research claims some people have a gene that causes a shortened sleep cycle while still allowing them to achieve a quality night's sleep without adverse effects.[34] If Mom wasn't one of those lucky ones, the ill effects could have contributed to Alzheimer's.

Mom would begin her day at our coffee station, adding creamer until her hot java became almost white then she'd meander about the kitchen chatting with the boys before they left for school. She loved to be a part of whatever they were doing and was always a willing spectator at their many sporting events. As with all of Mom's many grandkids, her love for my boys was unconditional, and they did no wrong in her eyes, even when they did in mine. She was intensely loyal, sometimes blindly so when it came to her kids and grandkids. Shortly after the boys left for school and just as she'd done at her home, Mom walked her dog to our local park or around parts of our neighborhood before breakfast. My neighbors grew accustomed to seeing this petite, friendly, white-haired lady and her little dog. She'd wave as she walked by, or better yet, stop and talk if someone dared set foot outside their door. That neighbor would often call me later and tell me they saw her, and I could always track her course by whoever called or texted.

She'd then return with a story about something or someone she encountered along the way: another friendly—or not—dog, garbage cans on the sidewalk that caused her to walk in the street, or, once, a neighbor who almost backed their car over her. After I heard all about her adventures, we would sit down to breakfast and then we'd head out for a day full of activities before the boys returned from school. Those were enjoyable visits, and we were always sad when spring approached and she'd make plans to return to Cincinnati.

Mom was four years old when the stock market crashed in 1929, triggering the Great Depression. Like many others in her generation, and because of those volatile and unstable times, she was raised with a strong work ethic. She was always busy when I was growing up and never stopped moving. Rarely did she sit down during the day, and she certainly didn't have any hobbies or leisure interests to break up the monotony. She was either working away from home or working at home. That was her life, and she expected all of us to bear our fair share from an early age although she shouldered the major burden. "Many hands make light work," was a frequent motto of hers, and that came directly from her mother.

She ran circles around me when I was young, and even into early adulthood. While I might have considered hard work being some aspect of intense physical fitness like running, swimming, or a grueling match of singles tennis, hers was true grit—the kind of physical labor that gets knees down and hands scrubbing toilets and floors. There were always tasks for us, growing up in a large family: something to be cleaned, laundry to be folded, meals to be prepped. I clearly remember wanting Mom to just sit and talk with me. I yearned for that, but there always seemed to be more to do and never enough time.

Mom continued that pattern of busyness when she came to visit, always insisting on helping. When she finally sat down, usually after dinner to watch TV, she would immediately nod off. When I suggested she head to bed because she was sleeping, her go-to response was always an adamant, "I am *not* sleeping, just resting my eyes!" Mom didn't want to miss a thing in life. Although Mom was never a participant on social media, the acronym FOMO—fear of missing out—perfectly describes the way she lived her life. Mom wanted to be a part of everything, everywhere—all the time. FOMO must have caused her to miss out on many ZZZs!

It might seem that someone who raised a large family and spent most of that time executing chores would be glad to have a break. That, however, was never the case. She had to keep her hands busy and had a peculiar addiction to doing laundry, beating a path to my laundry room every morning. I doubt my washer and dryer ever stopped cycling when she was in town. If there was a dish cloth used for more than a day or an item in the laundry basket, it was immediately washed alongside her nighties. Most days she also discovered something that required ironing. Often, after the boys left for school, she would venture into their bedrooms—a daunting mission reserved for the most daring of warriors of which I was not. Sometime later she'd emerge triumphantly from those dank and smelly chambers, announcing she'd made their beds and picked up their rooms, while proudly displaying a dirty sock or underwear found under their beds. Sometimes she would go into their closets, grab their permanent-press white uniform shirts that didn't require pressing, and march them off to the ironing board. Half a can of spray starch later those shirts could stand up by themselves! She loved to set the evening table in the morning after breakfast and always inquired about what we were having and how she could help with dinner's food prep.

I never understood Mom's insistence on working so hard when she didn't have to, but it seemed to be in her wiring. I had help with household chores and didn't need her to do anything. After she came to live with us, I just wanted her to relax, especially when I noticed her struggle with the little things she had always done unconsciously like peeling carrots, folding clothes, and setting the table. How could things so simple, that were once so easy, now be so hard?

Mom's diagnosis did change the way I treated her in that I didn't want her to push herself, but that is exactly how she lived her whole life, and if anything, she was more determined than ever to keep moving and help out. At times this was frustrating, especially when I wanted to get out the door and on with the day. Watching her methodically wash and dry coffee cups instead of stacking them in the dishwasher brought back memories of waiting on my toddlers to pick up their toys. I knew it was much easier and quicker to do it myself. Keys in hand and coat on, I'd step one foot out the door when she'd suggest we put out the supper plates. I really didn't think we needed to set the dinner table at 9 am, but, letting out a huge sigh, I would shut the door to the garage and quickly grab plates to help her place them.

She'd stare at me with the corners of her mouth drifting slightly downward every time I tried to help her out. Then she'd pause and her shoulders would shrug as it hit me, *I did it again—I rushed her.* Although I was just trying to move things along, Mom wasn't operating by my watch. Her world moved slower, and she lived much more in the moment than my often-self-imposed timeline allowed. She was losing so much, and I was focusing more on what she couldn't do or, at least, couldn't do as efficiently as I'd like. She only wanted to play a role and assist the bigger cause. Feeling useful not only improved her outlook, especially after her diagnosis, but, for her, hard work was simply a moral good. Staying busy was all she'd ever known.

I was watching Mom fold towels one day when I became captivated by her absorption in that dull activity. It offered an early glimpse into her collapsing world. Slowly folding one towel after another, she was smiling. She wasn't doing it the way she'd taught me as a child, the way she'd always done it, yet she appeared so peaceful and happy. It reminded me of my toddlers concentrating intensely when they became totally immersed in building Legos or assembling puzzles.

Observing her, I almost experienced envy, a peculiar feeling considering her condition. She didn't appear to be somewhere else in her mind as I often was while doing things. She was just there, serene, and certainly not the person I remembered always going a mile a minute. Alzheimer's might have muddled her thoughts, but it also allowed space between them—a rare thing for her. How could her mind which seemed so absent-minded at the same time allow her to be more present? I found myself wondering if I could be more like her in this way—more content and focused on the task at hand—just happy to be folding clothes or chopping carrots without my mind leaping ahead anxiously to something else. I had a fleeting thought that even in her dementia, Mom still had much to teach. Her happiness was enviable, but I certainly didn't want to discover this seemingly blissful state at the hands of dementia. So, how could I achieve it now?

This moment had still more to teach. Mom's demeanor changed whenever I gave her something to do by herself *and at her own pace.* Her ability to complete a task without being hurried brought about a positive transformation—a smile, and a little kick in her step! I understood then that her need to feel valued by helping equated to feeling loved. On a different level, that was something I could understand. I doubt helping with chores would do it for me, but I could relate to hungering for validation of dignity and love and the means I've sought to achieve it.

Mom wanted that too, and to be an important contributor she needed a daily mission. Retrieving smelly socks to be washed, peeling carrots, setting the table, or folding towels—however slow or imperfect these tasks looked to me—gained her entrance into the club. She was happy when helping and felt loved in the doing!

Alzheimer's robbed Mom of many things, but her desire to be significant and make a difference somewhere gave her a purpose, and that led to a very good day for everyone. It was early on in our journey with the disease, but if that's all it took, like Lou Gehrig said in his famous farewell speech at Yankee stadium, I was "the luckiest [woman] on the face of the earth."[35]

Chapter Sixteen

The Hostage Situation

Late Fall 2009

Gee Ma, I wanna go, but they won't let me go,
Gee Ma, I wanna go home.
Anonymous

The song, "Gee Mom I Want to Go Home," by an unknown author was originally written to satirize life in the Canadian Army during WWII. The above version came from the TV series *MASH*, but all versions depict individuals stuck in undesirable environments who long to return home. Mocking their circumstances with these lyrics brings comic relief. Mom developed her own adaptation and sang it every day—I WANT TO GO HOME—but, unlike the others, it brought no relief to either of us as she repeated it over and over. Just as I began to consider myself the least bit lucky with thoughts that Mom was acquiescing to her new living arrangement, the other shoe finally, unavoidably dropped—hard.

I kept the promises I made to Mom, and we enjoyed a summer and fall packed with weekend trips and day activities. She was in high spirits if she had something to look forward to and if we kept moving. Physical therapy was not one of her favorite things, but she got through it and soon her arm was functional again. That's when her long-term memories of her Cincinnati home reared their ugly head.

If Mom's body hadn't been so strong and healthy, she may have considered living with her daughter a welcomed respite. But her body had a mind of its own and was as strong-willed as she, defiantly pushing through falls, broken bones, and hip surgery up until her last years. After Dad passed, Mom kept busy, taking care of her home and dog, visiting family and friends, volunteering, travelling, golfing, walking, and, of course, shopping. She didn't have a device to track her steps, but I'll bet shopping alone secured many miles. In her late seventies she hiked parts of the Appalachian Trail in the North Georgia Mountains with us. In her early eighties she came along on several trails we hiked in the Canadian Rockies. In her mid-eighties she walked to our park almost daily, covering an arduous roller-coaster of a mile to the entrance. Once there, she continued a lap around the park before retracing those steps home.

She checked a lot of boxes when it came to possibly avoiding or delaying the onset of Alzheimer's: eating wholesome foods, getting plenty of exercise, and strong social interactions. This may have postponed the advent of her symptoms well beyond my grandmother's, but the latest research finds that active mental stimulation may be the best approach for delaying the onset: "Cognitively stimulating activities [lead] to changes in brain structure and function that enhance cognitive reserve. Repeated engagement in these activities may enhance certain neural systems so that relatively more harm is needed before they stop working."[36]

Although Mom was doing a lot of good things to stay healthy, her only mental stimulation was skimming the daily newspaper. She didn't have any hobbies that directly fueled her mind or could possibly induce positive changes in the brain like writing, knitting, taking new classes, puzzles, meditating, or learning a new language. She was always too busy for those things.

When she arrived in Atlanta with her broken arm, she was in the early stage of moderate decline or stage four out of seven on most charts that track the progression of Alzheimer's.[37] She was struggling with newly learned information, asking the same questions, and telling the same stories repeatedly. She could easily become irritated and frustrated and often had trouble articulating her ideas or finding the right words to express herself. Outside of physical assistance because of her arm, she needed oversight with medications and healthy food choices.

Even in stage four, it was difficult to pick up on her memory issues. Neighbors who didn't know of her diagnosis were very surprised after I told them. It was only after being with her for a while that her repetitions or other abnormalities became apparent, such as asking open-ended questions that required more thought processing than a simple yes or no.

When asked how she was, her go-to response was always, "Fine, and how are you?" When asked if she enjoyed seeing her great-granddaughter, she would respond with "Yes," and maybe even add, "She is darling." But if pressed further into the conversation and asked how old her great-granddaughter was, she would hesitate, and then retort, "Old enough." If asked if she liked the matinee from earlier that afternoon, she would reply yes or no. But if pushed on and asked about a character in the movie or what the movie was about, she would hesitate, and in that delay a veil spread over her eyes as her demeanor changed. Frustration set in and instead of answering the question asked, she would respond, "The movie was good,"—a hard-wired response that didn't require complex thought. Over time we realized that open-ended conversations were too painful for her, and equally painful for us to watch, so we tried to avoid them.

She was still trying to gloss over what she couldn't remember. It was a vicious cycle of forgetting, being aware of—and embarrassed by—that forgetfulness, then trying to cover it up. That usually resulted in an outburst of anger at me, which was totally out of character for her. In my estimation, stage four was the hardest for all of us as she still remembered much from her past.

When those memories returned, she just wanted to go home, often communicating plaintively to anyone who would listen, "BUT THEY WON'T LET ME GO."

Mom was diagnosed with MCI in Ohio around 2008 about a year before she came to live in Atlanta. After relocating her, we began working with a group of health care professionals in the neurology department at Emory University, initiating the process with a full neurological workup. This included medical history, a complete physical and neurological exam, mental status testing, and an MRI. The MRI revealed the small spots on Mom's brain were TIAs and had been occurring since midlife. She also exhibited shrinkage in different areas of her brain, especially the hippocampus. The diagnosis this time was Alzheimer's disease with vascular dementia. So, there it was—Alzheimer's—on paper in black and white.

A big part of me knew this before I read it. I had seen the pain and confusion in her eyes as she had tried to act as normal as possible, heard the frustration in her voice as she'd struggled with conversations, and I'd sensed in my heart her slipping ever so slowly . . . but until I'd read the clinical conclusion and spoken with the doctor, I could still have *some* hope, although I don't think my siblings had any. Mom was so physically strong that she could have lived to be a hundred—even while moderately confused—and I ruminated on that often. Until I received that report, I could still allow myself to believe that it was only MCI and that Mom wouldn't get much worse.

I've heard it said that serious diagnoses can sometimes bring relief as all the testing, wondering, and waiting for an explanation are finally over. A shift occurs as reality sets in—plans change, and dreams end at the period of a grim diagnostic report. Though the news was painful and sad, there was a strange kind of release in the knowing, a concession that opens the door to acceptance. There was no point in sharing this additional information with Mom, however, as she didn't accept the earlier diagnosis of MCI. Over a year later with continued memory loss, this information would only have brought more frustration and pain.

The recommendation was to continue Mom's treatment plan of the Exelon patch and a drug called Namenda, which were started in Ohio. These drugs cannot cure the disease but may temporarily pause the cognitive deterioration that allows activities such as bathing, eating, and dressing as well as language skills to remain where they are for a longer period.

❧❧❧

It was late fall when Mom's arm was fully functional and because she felt so good, she saw no reason to stay. That's when she launched the campaign to return home.

"I want to go home," she'd begin calmly. "I've been away long enough, and my house is sitting empty—I need to check on it." She'd then continue, and her rationale was sound. "My car hasn't been driven in so long, and the battery has probably run down."

Waiting for my response, she'd then begin to plead, "I really need to get back, Marianne, please let me go."

"Mom," I'd respond with a deep sigh, "We've been through this." I would then try to explain further, "Because you're having a hard time remembering important things, you can't live on your own, and you won't let anyone help you."

It was like she never heard anything I said, as she continued, "Well, I need to go home and take care of my home and car." And so it went, and usually downhill from there.

She was right about getting back and looking after her things, and, to an uninformed bystander, he made all the sense in the world—if she could only have remembered the correct day, to take her meds, or to turn off the water in her bathroom sink or the pot of carrots on the stove. She wasn't retaining newly learned information like how to use the TV remote or where the garage door button was located—even the microwave was beyond her comprehension.

Although she still remembered her life in Cincinnati and wanted it back, she didn't remember the reasons she was with me because she wasn't retaining those "last in" memories. Her most recent conversations didn't exist. If it wasn't a long-term, hard-wired memory, it was gone—evaporated. Unfortunately for both of us, her "first in" memories were well preserved. She remembered Cincinnati and her family and friends there whom she talked with on a regular basis, still plugging their numbers into the phone. But if asked about those conversations, she drew a frustrated blank.

In her mind, which at times seemed to pick and choose what she could remember, I was the single reason she remained trapped in Atlanta. I was the captor and she was the hostage. My hopes of an easy passage from remembering to forgetting her past disappeared on the brink of each new day as she steam-rolled her way into the kitchen, bringing with her memories of my grandmother stomping down the hall into my parents' kitchen. Ma's goal was food; Mom's goal was freedom. Her song, "I want to go home, I want to go home, I want to go home!" became her daily and unrelenting battle cry.

Chapter Seventeen

The Bad Guy

April 2010

When you come to the end of your rope, tie a knot and hang on.
Franklin D. Roosevelt

"Mom, you just ate the dog's food!" Cathy exclaimed as Mom nibbled away at the kibbles in a bowl on the kitchen counter.

"Well, it tastes just like all of the other garbage she feeds me!"

It was Holy Thursday and much of Mom's extended family had travelled from Ohio and Florida to celebrate Easter with us. I set out an assortment of appetizers on the kitchen island as the family gathered around to reconnect and unwind. Probably excited about the party atmosphere and possibly overwhelmed at the same time, she confused the dog food on the counter with the spread of appetizers and happily munched away.

Her snipe about my culinary skills as well as her inability to distinguish dog and human food spoke volumes about the degree of cognitive decline she had experienced since her move to Atlanta the previous summer. Mom's remark signaled not only her discontent with her living arrangements but also her exasperation with me. As is the case with many caregivers, I became the focus of her anger and frustration—I was the bad guy. By no fault of her own, and within a year's time, she had lost control over the direction of her life. She now lived with my family five hundred miles away from other family and friends, ate what I prepared, went where I went because she was not driving, and saw who I saw. Naturally, she associated me with the loss of the life she'd known.

This was extremely painful because, before Alzheimer's, she had always loved being with me. The irony was, she'd enjoyed all those things when they were her choice, but that option vanished when she began battling this brain-pilfering beast. Now, in her mind, I was the roadblock to that old life and independence. I was a wall to be torn down, and she was doing a bang-up job of it. Slowly but surely, I was crumbling.

Even with a rational and reasonable mind, it is difficult to submit and surrender to the adversities in life that bring change. When a loved one dies, when we lose our job, get divorced, or experience mental or physical illness within ourselves or our families, our life's course is thrown off. Even happy milestones like a child graduating high school and leaving for college can trigger the blues, a foreshadowing of separation that screams, "Your life is about to change, and you're not going to like it!"

A lot of the changes that occur during our earthly existence are normal and healthy—just part of the plan—although they still hurt as we ride the emotional roller coaster we call life. I've heard it said that most emotions last ninety seconds and beyond that it's a choice of whether we remain there or not. Many experts in the mental health field believe it's best to ride those emotions out like a wave as they swell, break, and recede. We feel what comes up, let it break us—however that looks—and then let it slowly subside.

This would have been helpful information when Mom was in the early throes of her disease—when she was combative and when my anger and frustration, whether I expressed it or not, boiled up and lingered longer than hers did because I couldn't forget. Although it felt like I was fighting Mom or she was fighting me, the reality was that we were both wrestling with the beast called Alzheimer's as it rammed change down our throats like no other.

Mom's need to control her life made sense, especially because she didn't have the ability to comprehend why it had been upended so drastically. She was grieving a life well before it ended and couldn't work through her emotions in a healthy or logical way. So, she dealt with the chaos through hostility and outbursts, which were an indicator of the frustration of her loss. Those doggone memories of 3490 Highfields Lane kept coming back without the more recent details that explained the whys of her departure. Her "fading brain" didn't allow her a chance of comprehending any of this.

I couldn't explain something that left no imprint on her brain, but I still tried out of sheer exasperation. I said it plenty when my kids were young, but "Because I said so" never felt like something I should ever say to my mom. Trust me though, that phrase was often on the tip of my tongue as I heard her continual "Why can't I go home?" After explaining for the hundredth time why she couldn't go home, I'd try to ignore her and go about my business, thinking she would eventually get tired of asking, but that was like pouring gasoline on the never-extinguished embers burning within her. Then, everything went up in flames. In anger she'd lash out, "I am your mother, and you can't keep me here, I want you to take me home—NOW!" She wasn't alone in that desire because I really wished I could take her home—or anywhere else but there—in those moments. She'd retreat into her bedroom. Her resulting vexation was shorter lived than mine as she quickly forgot most every conversation. Meanwhile, as I was taking deep breaths and talking myself off the cliff, I would hear her stomping through the family room into the kitchen or wherever I might be. She'd square up against me, and the protests to go home would begin anew. "Mom . . ." I'd respond with a deep sigh.

It was an endless loop and a no-win for either of us. I knew better than to go down that road, and, when I did, lingering remorse for continuing a circular dialogue or ignoring her altogether established residence in me. I knew trying to reason with her was senseless, and it brought back memories of Mom doing the same thing with my grandmother, although she had a viable excuse because Mom knew virtually nothing about the disease then.

I echoed the frustrations of Paul in Romans 7:15 when he said, "I do not understand what I do. For what I want to do I do not do, but what I hate I do." Nothing short of going home would stop Mom's nostalgia, and that was the cruelty of late stage four, remembering the good old days without the memory to function in them.

Unlike Mom, I had breathers. I could talk it out in support groups with others ahead of me on the same road and vent with family and friends. I briefly escaped Alzheimer's by going for a swim, taking a solo walk, or meditating. I was dealing with a disease that was affecting my mom's brain, but there were days when I thought I was the one losing my mind. I constantly reminded myself that someone had to stay calm and reasonable.

I often wondered if Mom dreamt about home in her sleep because mornings were her most aggressive time of day. She woke up ready to fight, whereas in the evenings she was more agreeable. So, just like finding ways to distract my toddlers when they wanted something they couldn't have, I had to divert Mom's attention from wanting to going home. Instead of answering her hostility with more, I realized there was a way to reroute her attention. Like my dog when I mention the word *treat*, Mom's new buzzword was *shopping*! I began to use this tactic daily, and soon I was an expert at devising ways to make everyday errands sound like a trip to Disney World or at least Northpoint Mall.

At the Fresh Market she could pour herself a cup of flavored coffee, adding a heap of natural sugar and lots of cream, while strolling the store checking out fresh fish, assorted produce, and mounds of coffee beans from all corners of the world. I had to closely watch her because she thought the large clear bins of nuts and candies were free samples. More than once, while I was off gathering items, I would find her dispensing an enormous quantity of jellybeans or M&Ms into her hand, which then quickly overflowed onto the floor.

Costco and Sam's Club were other favorites. There, she could wander around the store independently with her own cart, sample the numerous tastings offered, and browse the clothing sections. She always came away with an item or two of women's apparel that she "absolutely needed" in her wardrobe or that she thought I needed in mine. Besides clothing, her basket usually held a few sweets and sometimes a toy for her great-granddaughter.

After completing my checklist of items, I would swing around to collect her. I always found her chatting with someone—the lady serving samples of cheese and crackers, the gentleman trying to sell her a Ninja blender, or the sweet, unsuspecting mom with small kids patiently listening to her talk about having lunch with Barbara Bush. She thrived on these outings where she had a chance to roam the aisles at her own pace, talk with people, and share her stories. Social interactions were nearly as vital to her as the air she breathed.

Her favorite distraction was also my worst nightmare—a trip to the mall. I did it though because watching Mom try on clothing for hours was a whole lot better than listening to her rant about going home. Even in this stage, Mom could lose hours as she shopped for clothing she didn't need. She never forgot her love of fashion, and shopping filled a void that had surfaced after my dad died. To deal with her ongoing grief at that time, she began meeting with her parish priest on a regular basis. She always got a kick out of repeating a conversation where Father told her to distract herself by doing something she loved. She told him she loved shopping, so he told her to shop, and she did. Spending hours in a store became a pastime that never ended precisely because, in her words, "He never told me when to stop!"

I was still the bad guy, mostly in the mornings, but if I could run her around enough during the day, she was too tired to remember and argue at night. Tying a knot at the end of my rope and holding on during Mom's worst moments helped me make it through another day!

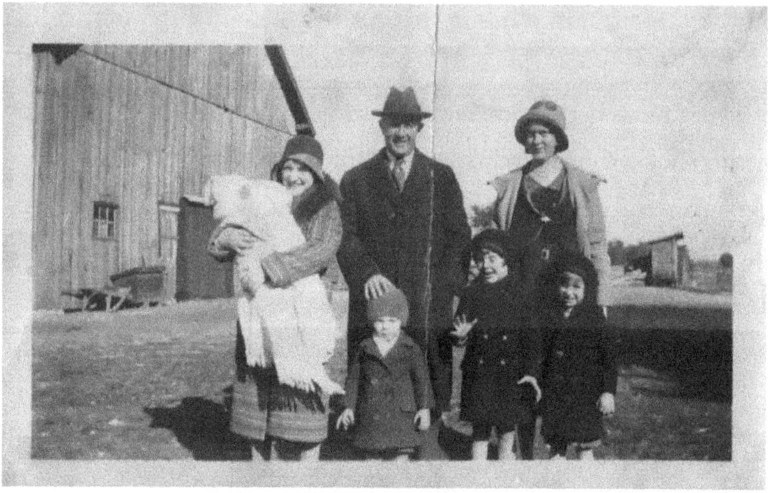

Image 1. My grandmother's family. *Front row, left to right:* Mom and her other siblings. *Back row, left to right:* Ma holding her son Donnie, Pa, unknown. Ohio, 1930s.

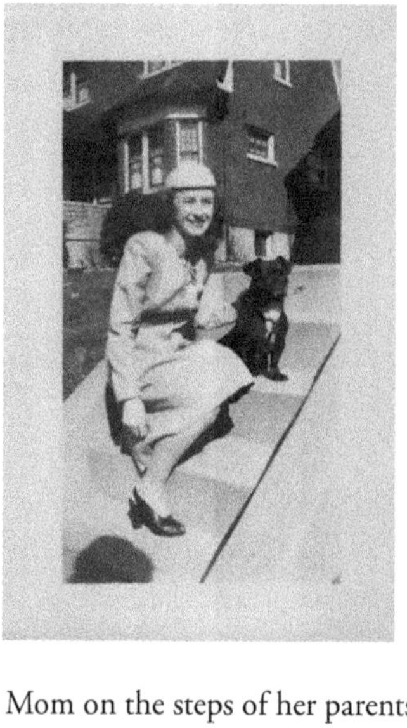

Image 2. Mom on the steps of her parents' home. Amberley Village, Ohio, circa 1943.

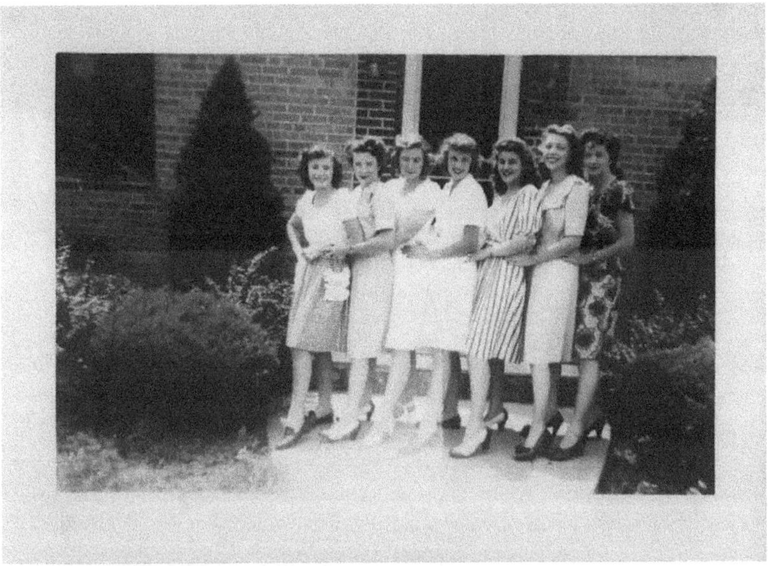

Image 3. Mom, her cousin, and many of her girlfriends who became like family. Ohio, circa 1944.

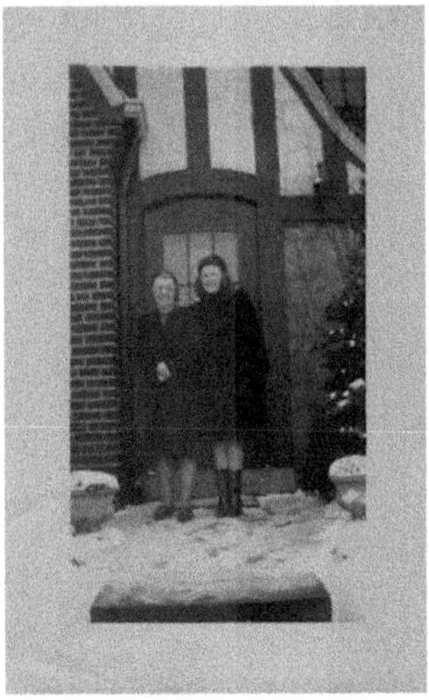

Image 4. Ma and Mom on the front steps of my grandparents' home. Amberley Village, Ohio, circa 1946.

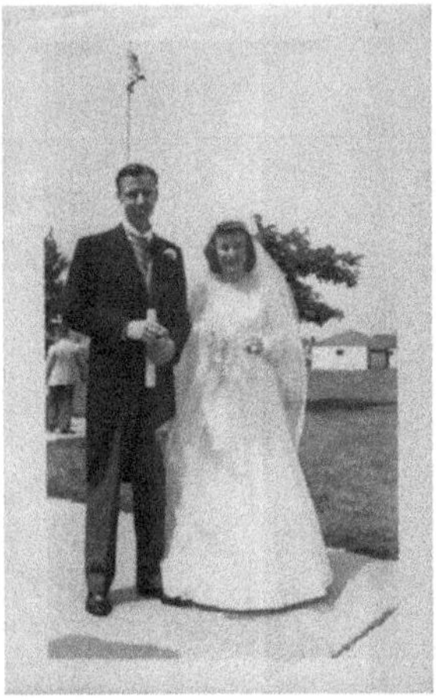

Image 5. Mom and Dad on their wedding day. Cincinnati, Ohio, 1948.

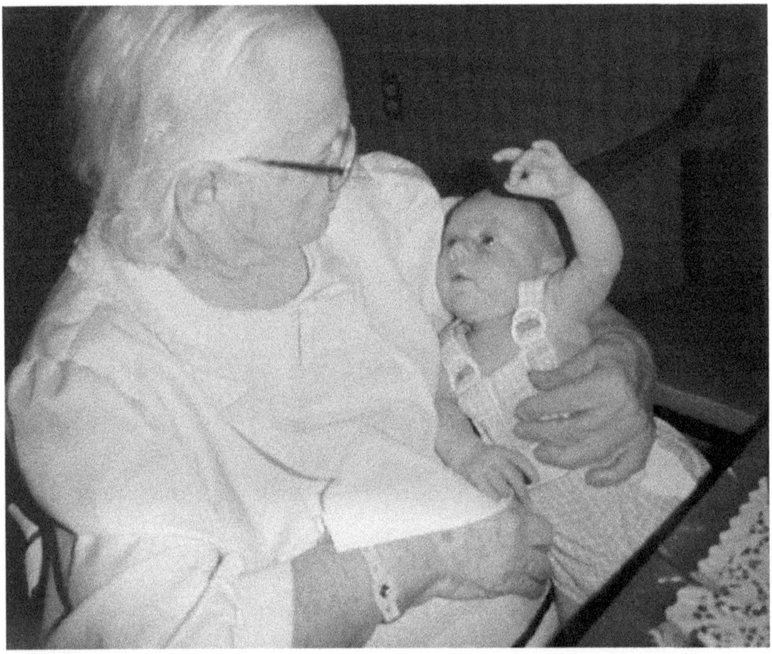

Image 6. Ma holding my oldest child, Ryan. Ohio, circa 1986.

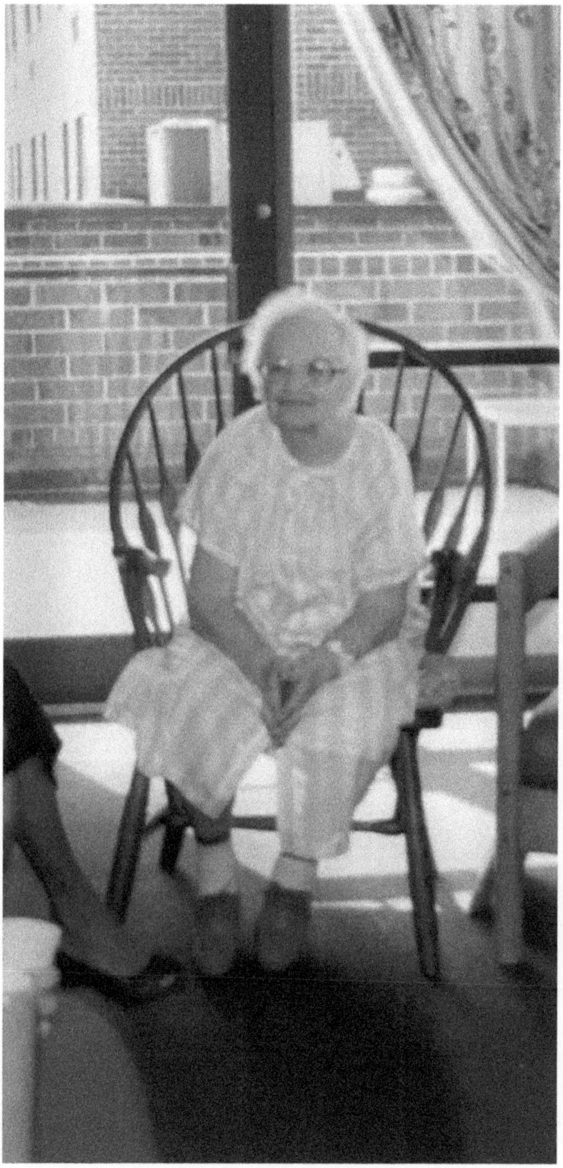

Image 7. Ma in a common area of her nursing unit. Cincinnati, Ohio, circa 1989.

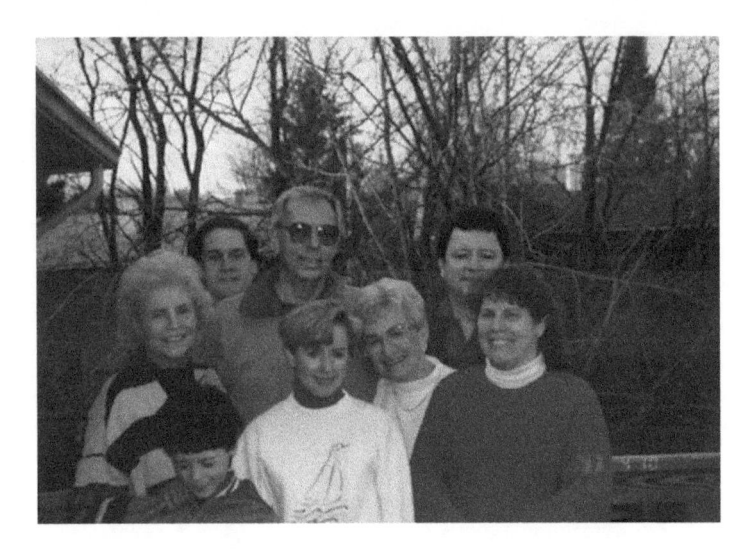

Image 8. *Front row, left to right:* My Aunt Mogie, my nephew Colin, me, Mom, my sister-in-law Margaret. *Back row, left to right:* My husband Steve, Dad, my brother Pat. Cincinnati, Ohio circa 1993.

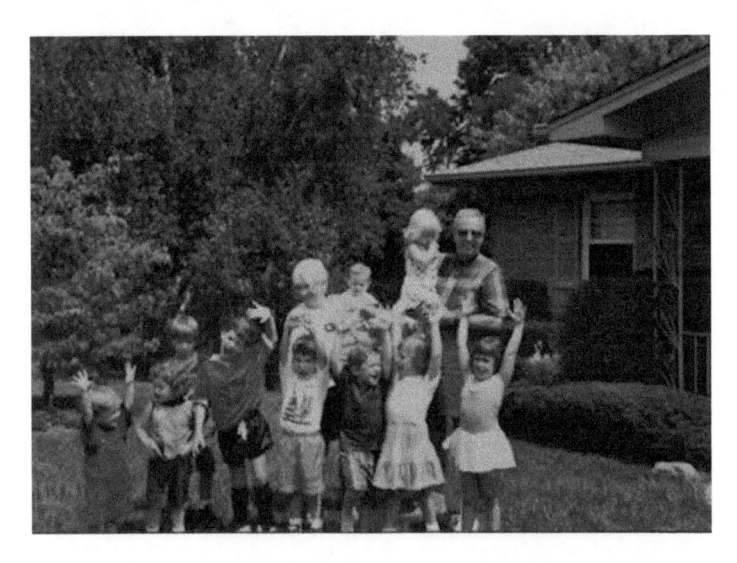

Image 9. Mom and Dad in front of their home with many of their grandkids. Cincinnati, Ohio, circa 1994.

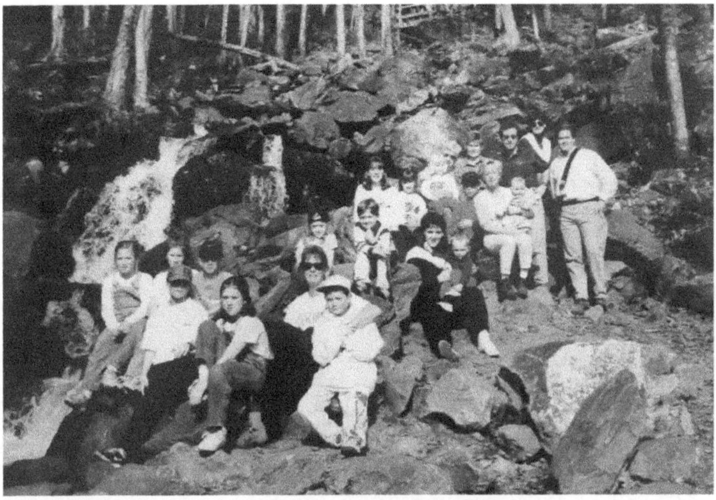

Image 10. Mom, right back row holding a grandchild, after a family hike. Amicalola Falls in the North Georgia Mountains, circa 1997.

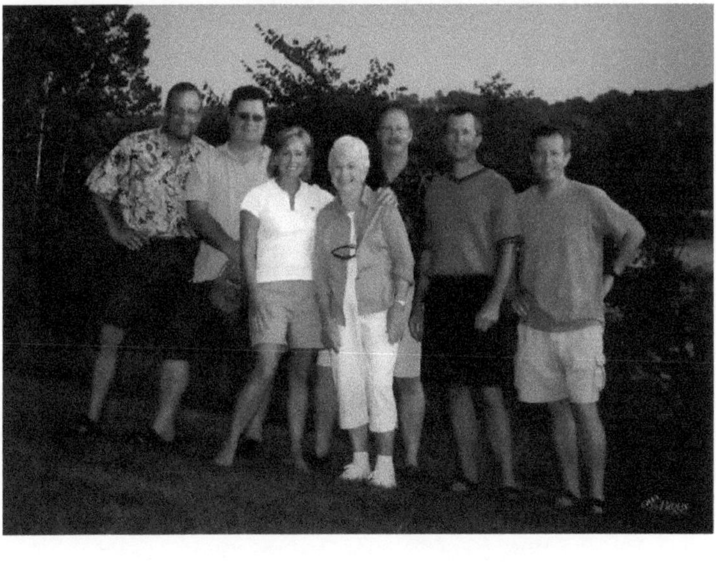

Image 11. Mom with all her children. *Left to right:* Joe, Pat, me, Mom, Mike, Kevin, Tim. Ohio, circa 2004.

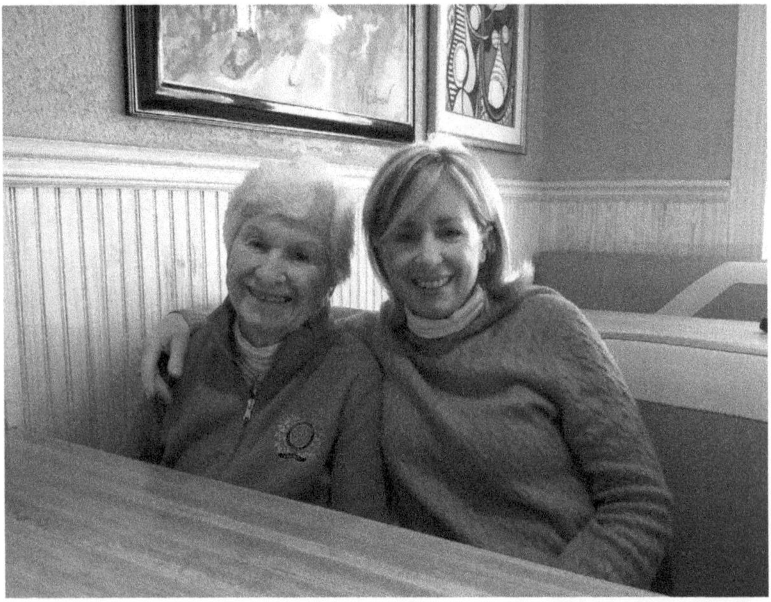

Image 12. Mom and I at a restaurant shortly after her move to my home. Alpharetta, Georgia, circa 2009.

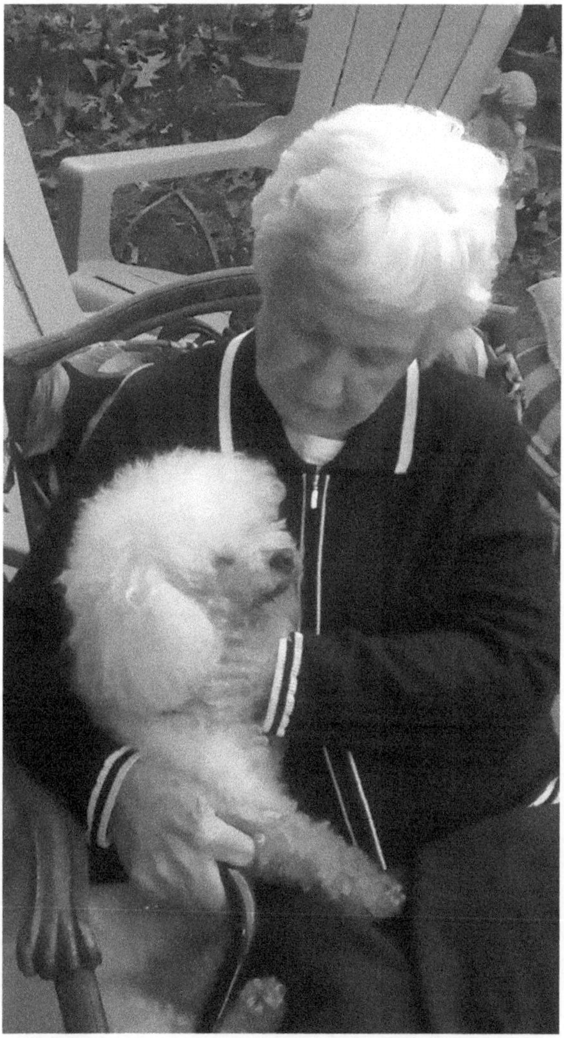

Image 13. Mom holding her beloved Abby at our home. Alpharetta, Georgia, circa 2009.

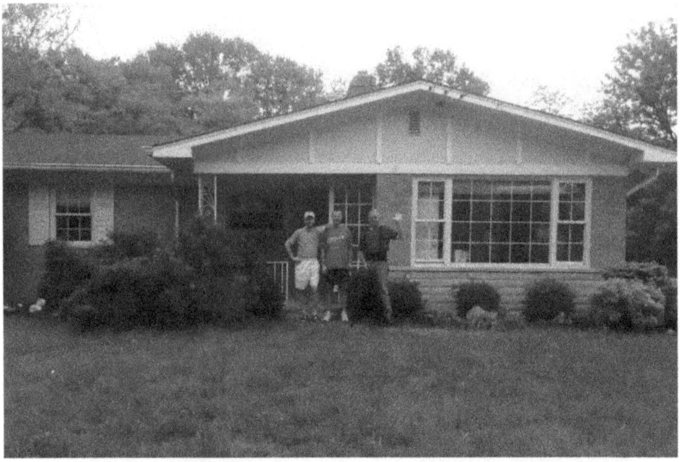

Image 14. My brothers (*left to right:* Tim, Kevin, and Joe), in a final picture in front of our childhood home after making it ready for its new owners. Cincinnati, Ohio, circa 2010.

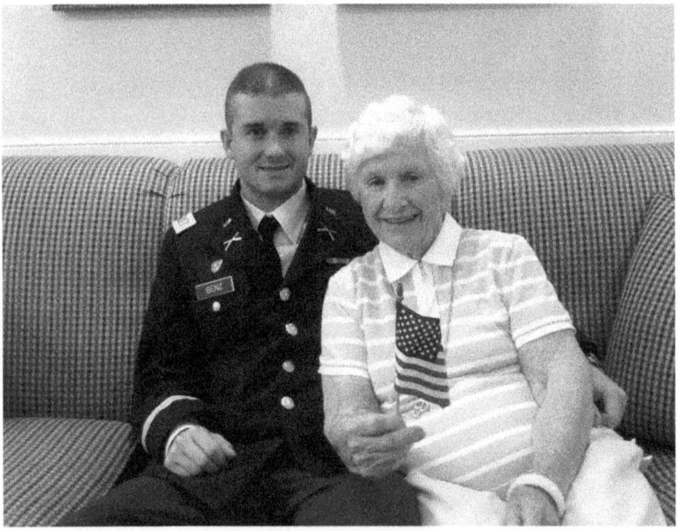

Image 15. My son, Ryan, during a visit home, with Mom in assisted living. Alpharetta, Georgia, circa 2010.

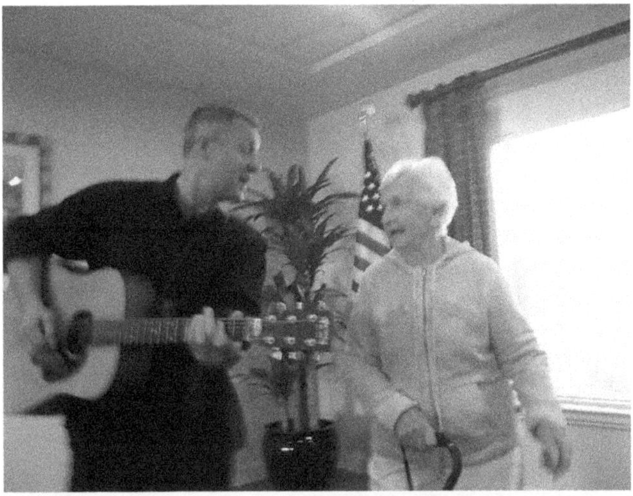

Image 16. Mom boogying to the entertainment in assisted living. Alpharetta, Georgia, circa 2011.

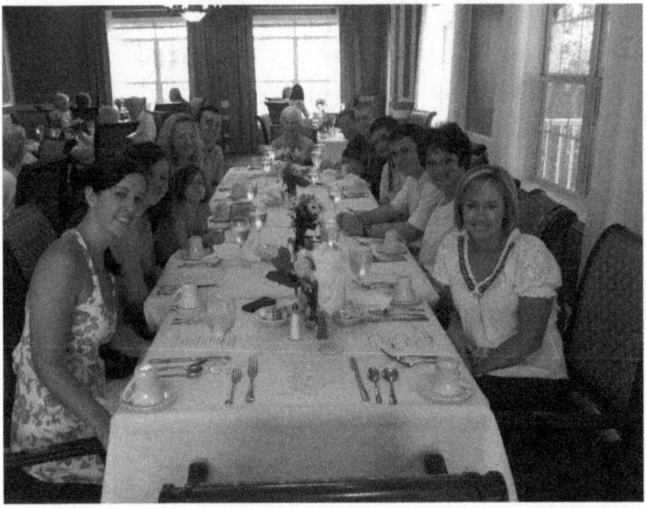

Image 17. Many of Mom's kids having dinner in the restaurant in the independent living section of her retirement community. Alpharetta, Georgia, circa 2011.

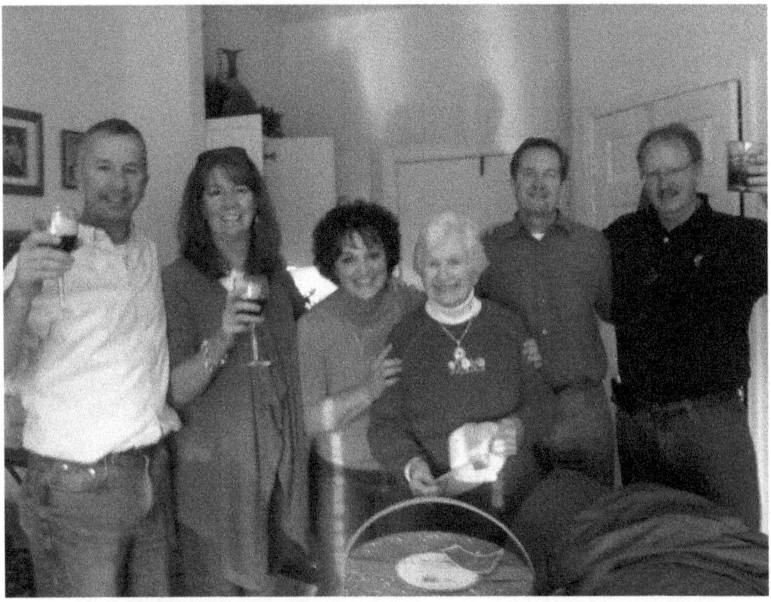

Image 18. *Left to right:* Kevin, Charlyne, Kathy, Mom, Steve, and Mike. Part of the Christmas decorating crew during a Thanksgiving weekend. Alpharetta, Georgia, circa 2011.

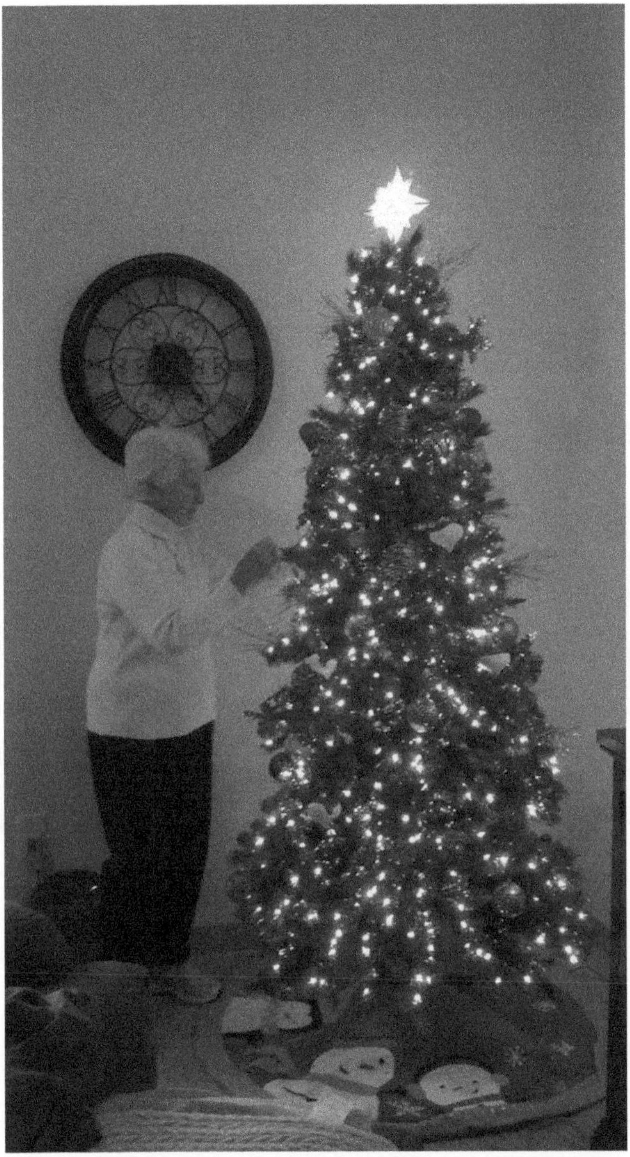

Image 19. *The final touch*, a representation of the treasured *Red Bird* that Mom saw everywhere after Dad's death. Alpharetta, Georgia, circa 2011.

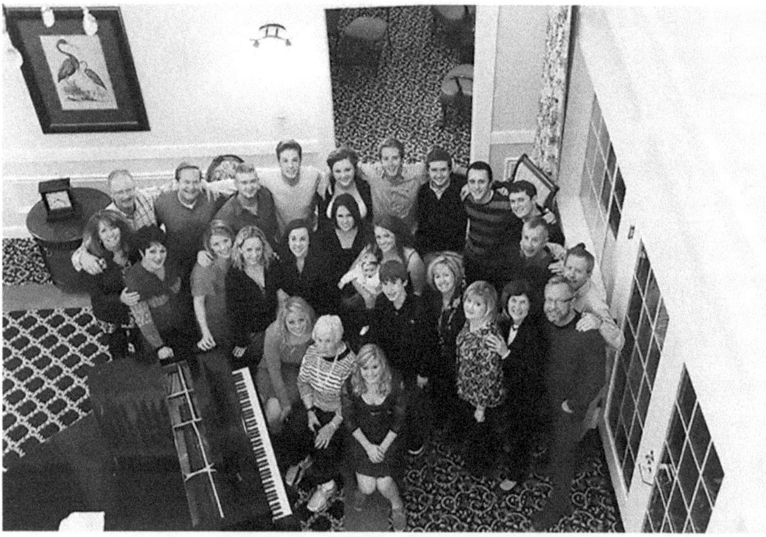

Image 20. Celebrating Mom's birthday in assisted living with extended family. Alpharetta, Georgia, circa 2012.

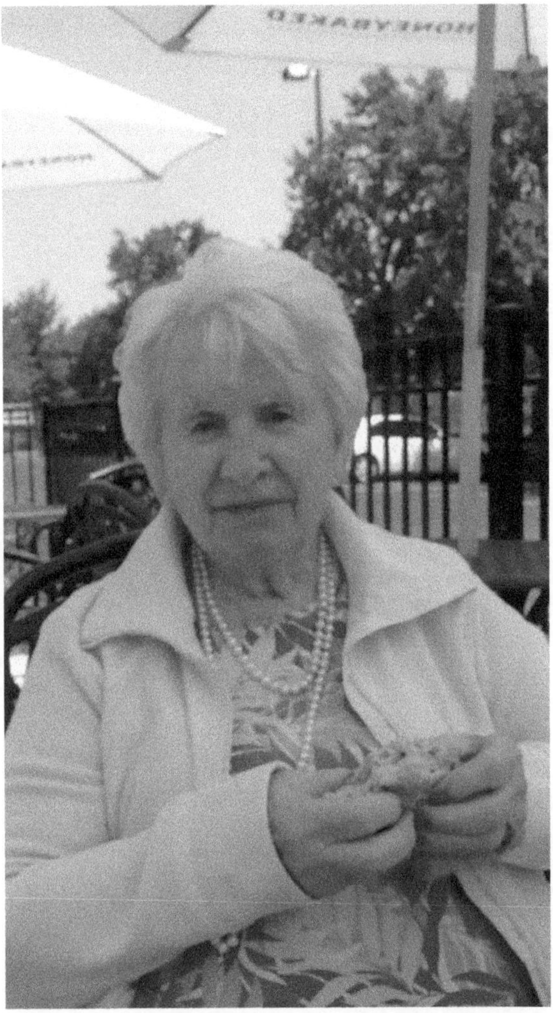

Image 21. Mom having lunch with me outside Honey Baked Ham during her time in assisted living. Alpharetta, Georgia, circa 2012.

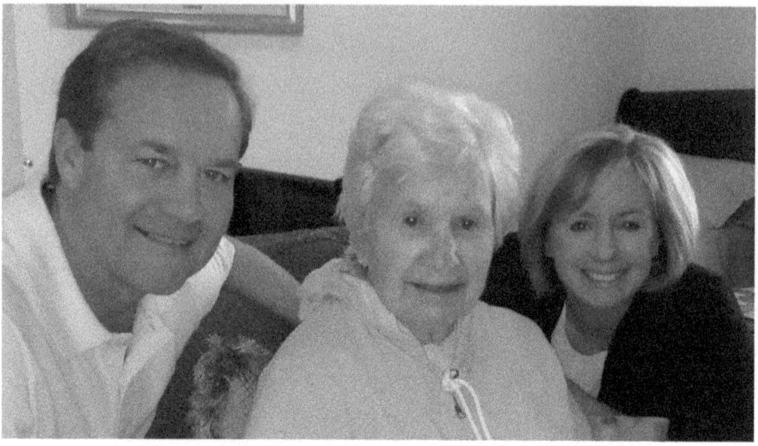

Image 22. Steve, Mom, and I in her assisted living room. Alpharetta, Georgia, circa 2012.

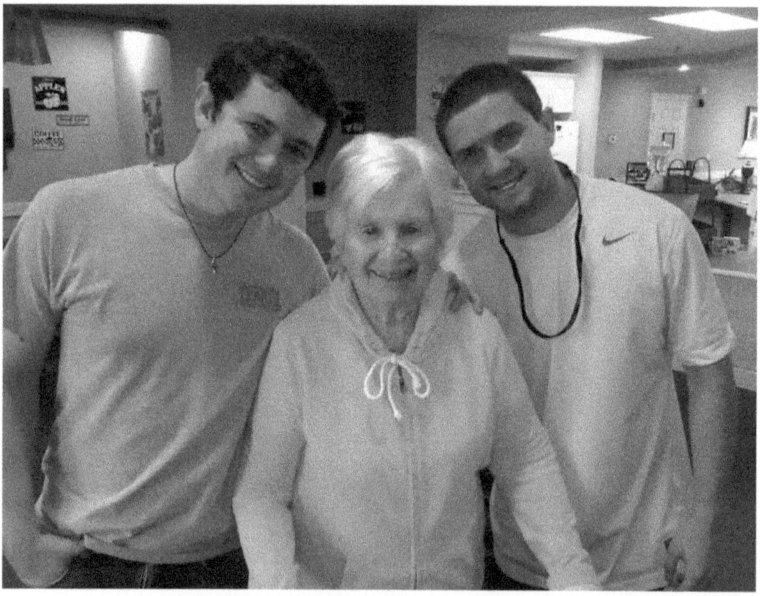

Image 23. My sons, Brady and Drew, with Mom in memory care. Alpharetta, Georgia, circa 2013.

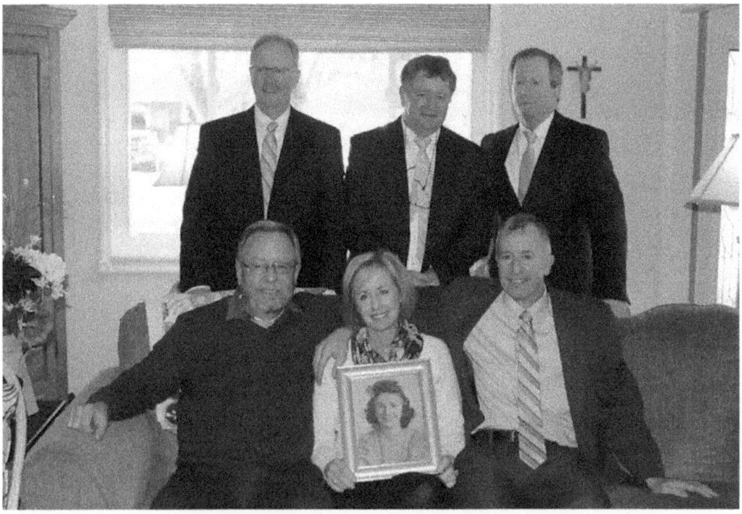

Image 24. My siblings and I at Mom's wake with her picture at Kevin and Cathy's home. Cincinnati, Ohio, January 2015.

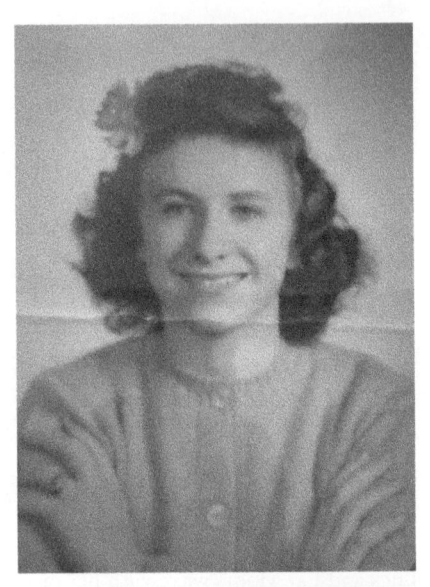

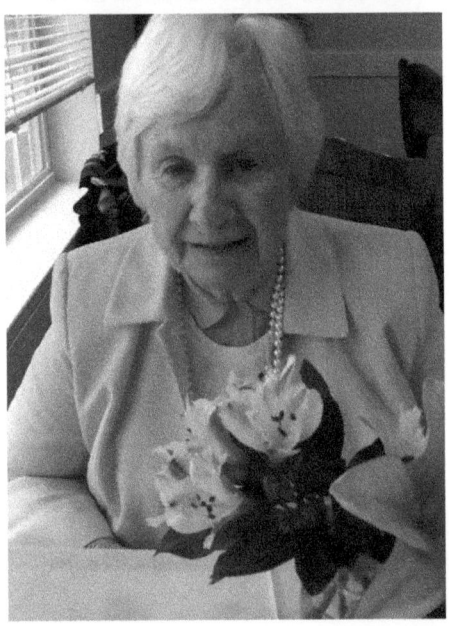

Images 25 and 26. Mom, circa 1945 and circa 2012.

Chapter Eighteen

Call in the Troops

There must be those among us with whom we can sit down and weep and still be counted as warriors.
ADRIENNE RICH

We live in a culture where vulnerability is frowned upon, and we don't want to be viewed as weak. I grew up believing the stronger I appeared emotionally and intellectually, the more I would be accepted and loved. I didn't feel that pressure coming from my parents because it was self-inflicted. I had to be in control or I could make a mistake or even fail.

This flawed approach to life causes a lot of unnecessary stress, and it certainly didn't work well with Alzheimer's. Becoming educated around Alzheimer's was important, but thinking I could control this disease and hold my emotions in led to much anxiety and even depression.

A few months after Mom came to live with us, and after her Alzheimer's diagnosis, I joined a local support group for Alzheimer's and dementia caregivers, which I found through the National Institute on Aging. They directed me, through the Alzheimer's Association, to a nearby church group that met on Wednesday mornings. Later, I joined another group that met at a nearby retirement community. These groups became my oxygen as I navigated the complex and ever-changing world of Alzheimer's. This disease is progressive and has many moving parts: medical, psychological, physical, emotional, spiritual, and legal. Just when I felt comfortable, something would change, causing a new challenge to arise, and we were back to the drawing board.

One of the groups I attended was facilitated by a nurse who was well-versed in most areas of dementia. The meeting was held in a small office, just down the hall from the narthex of the church. On my initial visit, everyone was seated around the large table when I entered the room, but the warm smiles that greeted me as I walked in calmed my nerves and put me at ease. I looked around at the group, quickly realizing I was the youngest attendee. This was my first experience with any type of support group, and I was nervous. But as everyone looked up as I walked in, offering warm smiles, my shoulders relaxed and I felt at ease. I also experienced a sense of security—like being with my dad—as I realized the years of experience gathered around that table would provide much needed guidance and support. Those assembled consisted of caregivers of all ages and genders but mostly over fifty. There were also individuals whose loved one had passed and who just came to share their wisdom.

Call in the Troops

I sat silently as others shared their pain and stories, and, for the first time since Mom was diagnosed, I felt less alone on my journey and safe enough to let my guard down. I still remember the enormous weight lifted from my shoulders when I told our story to this group of total strangers. Their collective nods and compassionate expressions encouraged me, giving me the nerve to release everything I had been holding so tightly.

One comment made by a gentleman at my very first meeting, about a reality that characterized the progressive nature of Alzheimer's, left an imprint that proved its truth again and again. He remarked that the frustration and angst Mom was experiencing would slowly get better with time. His words guided my course of action moving forward, which made the tough decisions somewhat easier. A simple observation, but within it was the hidden paradox of the disease: Mom's inner turmoil would get better by her cognition getting worse.

I gleaned so much from this group. Outside of advice and tips, I found emotional solace from my own mental anguish, feelings that ran the gamut from grief to guilt. The grief is ongoing, losing a loved one bit by bit, and the guilt comes from many different angles. For me it was making challenging decisions that ran counter to what Mom would have wanted, decisions that were necessary but still haunted me at night.

These support groups were also a treasure trove of information for resources in my area. I learned about home health care companies and what they provided—a wide range of services covering everything from simple companionship to full nursing care as well as physical, occupational, and speech therapy all within the home. I listened to reviews and recommendations of nearby retirement communities with assisted living, memory care, and full nursing facilities. I also received the names of reputable elder care attorneys, who serve as advocates for elderly and disabled individuals.[38] Elder care attorneys specialize in family trusts, estate planning, durable and medical powers of attorney, legal guardianship, and advance directives. I also learned the hard way that there are numerous types of trusts that accommodate different situations, so do your homework, or, like us, run the risk of having to break down the first trust to set up a second.

My dad served in WWII, and an older gentleman in one of the support groups had told about a little-known secret for veteran benefits. Mom, as a surviving spouse of a veteran, was entitled to a monthly pension benefit under the Veteran's Administration Aid and Attendance Program. This program is set up for the veteran or their spouse who requires the aid and assistance of another person whether they live alone or in assisted living or memory care facilities. The monthly payment from this program is meant to help offset the costs involved in caring for someone who can't care for themselves due to many different reasons. Mom was eventually awarded this pension but not without the assistance of an attorney due to the complex and time-consuming applications and administrative tasks. There are, however, elder care attorneys in most areas who provide pro bono legal help for families and individuals who cannot afford their services.

What made our situation extra complicated was that we had no record of Dad's military service and discharge papers as they had been lost in the 1973 fire at the National Personnel Records Center in St. Louis. That fire destroyed most of the records of Army veterans discharged from 1912 to 1960. Luckily though, a family member suggested we check with the local county courthouse where Dad had lived when he was discharged. Sure enough, upon returning from war, my dad registered his discharge papers with the Hamilton County Courthouse, so we were able to verify his service. This process did take the better part of a year, largely due to securing Dad's military records, but the payments were retroactive back to the date of the application, and the financial reward was well worth the effort.

A member of my support group recommended engaging a geriatrician instead of a primary care doctor for Mom. Geriatrics is a specialty of internal medicine that encompasses all the conditions that affect the elderly rather than a specific area of the body or disorder. I had a hard time finding one, and some only accept a certain number of Medicare patients in their practice, but that also was well worth the time and effort.

After going through the selection process, I now consider geriatrics more of a calling than a job. Mom's doctor was not only well-versed in dementia but also compassionate and attuned to treating the whole person instead of just a symptom. Letting Mom try to explain her ailment or what she was feeling was a painful process to witness, but her doctor always gave Mom the first chance to talk. That opportunity must have validated Mom as a person because, even as she struggled, she still tried hard to express what must have been bottled up inside.

My support groups were a lifeline during some of our more difficult days, and I am grateful to have met some incredibly evolved souls. The most important things I learned went beyond tips, suggestions, and information to philosophies that aided me then and in my work as a hospice volunteer today.

I learned it's OK to have bad days and not feel the need to sugarcoat things or be stoic. I discovered it's OK to acknowledge nothing will ever be the same and admit that sometimes life just sucks and it might just suck until it doesn't. I realized it's OK to make mistakes along the way and not feel bad about them, but instead, to recognize when love drove those decisions and to dwell there—mistakes are not failure. I learned it's not just OK but vital to spend time every day in activities that clear my mind and support my body, so I can have a chance of responding instead of reacting to difficult situations. And I learned it's not OK or healthy to rush loss but better instead to feel it, and when I found myself missing that person standing right in front of me, I found it's OK to weep.

Dust and dirt were spinning around us in a cataclysmic vacuum of struggle and loss, and sometimes that's all I could see. But, occasionally, the sun's rays broke through, taking the form of beleaguered warriors who shared the arduous path with me. God's grace sprang forth from that dirt as I was beginning to learn. Henri Vaughn framed this up beautifully in his poem, "The Revival," "And here in dust and dirt, Oh here [/] The lilies of His love appear!"[39]

Chapter Nineteen

The Tough Decision

Spring 2010

In any moment of decision, the best thing you can do is the right thing, the next best thing is the wrong thing, and the worst thing you can do is nothing.
Theodore Roosevelt

As Mom's disease progressed, I employed a home health care company owned by a neighborhood friend. The services she offered were varied, but I chose the lowest level of care—more visiting friend than visiting nurse service. A few days a week, several hours a day, someone, usually the same person, would take Mom on an outing. I knew most of these ladies from the neighborhood or church, so I was comfortable with them and knew Mom was in good hands. I always informed Mom ahead of the visit that her friend was coming to see her.

Initially skeptical, after a few of these excursions, she readily set off with them. They would have lunch out then go shopping, to movies, a museum, or a walk around the park. Mom grew to love these daytrips and especially enjoyed the company of these friendly and caring women. They lavished attention on her, and I savored the break. By the time they returned, she was tired from a long afternoon, and I was refreshed and ready to resume caregiving.

I used this service until Mom became too challenging for the caregivers. For example, Mom always carried money in her purse and the caregiver had my credit card. Mom could buy whatever she wanted, but, at some point, she started shoplifting small items and not necessarily anything she needed or wanted—just random things she could easily pick up and conceal in her coat pocket or purse. When confronted, she would become indignant, stubbornly insisting she'd paid and refusing to relinquish the stolen goods. Luckily, the store employees were compassionate after being told of Mom's condition and her caregiver would pay without any legal actions taken. A cogent Mom would have been outright appalled by her "criminal" behavior but for the Alzheimer's silver lining: she never remembered her thievery.

Did I mention Mom was stubborn? Just like my toddlers who never wanted to leave the park or pool, Mom became defiant with her caregiver when she didn't want to leave a place, especially when they were shopping. She was quickly becoming a handful, and these sweet ladies couldn't pick her up and put her in the car as they might with a small child. This type of home health care was the lowest level provided, and Mom soon exhausted it as well as the "friends" who came to take her out.

After home health care fell through, I tried a couple of adult day centers designed for individuals with dementia. These programs offer structured activities in a group setting that gave the guest a chance to interact with their peers. I started Mom in half-day mornings, but, after a few weeks, she still wasn't joining in. She was spending most of the day walking to the front door, being redirected, and ending up back at the door again.

We'd told Mom that living with us was temporary until her arm healed. As her only daughter I always knew I would take Mom if she became unable to care for herself. I had the room, time, and resources, and to do otherwise went against everything I believed and had promised. Even though I lived at home after my grandmother was diagnosed, I looked on as a bystander as Mom bore the brunt of that responsibility. I knew keeping Mom would be challenging, but I had no idea of the impact full-time caregiving for a dementia patient would have on me and my mental health. It was reaching the point where something would have to give.

There was also a huge disparity between Mom's and Ma's attitude regarding independence. My grandmother feared being alone and wanted nothing more than to live out her life with our family, but Mom was desperate to return to her own home. This irony didn't escape me, especially as she voiced that sentiment increasingly and acrimoniously over the latter part of the year she spent with me. We were both miserable.

Although Mom could still be distracted, these shifts were only Band-Aids that momentarily paused her torment and outbursts. We were riding a slowly ascending roller coaster that lingered at the top of the track just long enough for us to catch our breath then plunged downward at warp speed. In front of us was always another hill.

Despite these difficulties, there were days when I couldn't bear the thought of her living somewhere else—not only because she couldn't care for herself and would be a lot for any facility to handle but also because I'd promised Mom I would never leave her anywhere she didn't want to be. This internal conflict was eating away the time I had left with her. She couldn't leave, but she also couldn't stay. She didn't want to live with me because her brain was running clips of her home, her car, and her life in Cincinnati. Every time these replayed, it stole her peace from the present. With a coherent mind, she would have chosen me, but she wasn't running the show.

Many days I couldn't wait for night to fall, just to escape her negativity and confrontation. It was beyond heartbreaking when someone I loved, and who I knew loved me, said awful things about me, and I found myself wanting to say awful things back. Sleep was a reprieve for both of us. Upon awakening I'd meditate in those quiet, early moments, trying to imagine Mom's pain and place myself in her hurt and confusion. Then I'd pray she'd sleep in for a few hours and for the grace to handle yet another day. I'd join my husband in the kitchen and prepare my tea. In these moments calm reigned.

The Tough Decision

Despite the stress, I was good to go, or so I thought. Then I would cringe as I heard the pitter patter of her slippers on the hardwood floors as she made her way across the house and into the kitchen, a little after six each morning. Even before getting coffee, she started her talk-track of wanting to go home, and my equanimity slowly evaporated. Mom was in her eighties with a brain-deteriorating disease, and I didn't want to squander the limited time I had with her fighting. I wasn't just battling Alzheimer's; I was at war with my myself, my guilt, my unwavering commitment to Mom, and my desire to be free of her daily care. Normally a positive person, I couldn't seem to overcome my increasing negativity about the situation, and moments of peace were short lived. My husband was my receptacle and my rock as he listened to me rant and watched me cry until I realized that my venting had become an end it itself—I wasn't accomplishing anything productive.

I didn't see a creative solution as I couldn't live with my mom, not like this, yet I couldn't live with myself if I moved her elsewhere. She was an innocent victim, and that's what really stung. There was no one to blame, and nowhere to unload the miserable situation. I was in a dark tunnel with no light in sight as I expressed in my writings from that period. I finally understood the reason for and extent of Mom's conflict with herself when she moved my grandmother from our home. Decades apart, we were fighting the same war.

I was still raising a family and running a business out of my home while spending the day with Mom. I could have hired someone to come and help with her, but that would not have stopped her mental discontent, and likely would have added to the tension. I was mentally and emotionally at my limit. She was up early, didn't nap, and didn't go to bed until we did. Her excessive amount of energy was further driven by her inner anguish, and her constant badgering wore me down.

Remaining sane was an objective but not my only one. I also wanted to live out Mom's journey with some semblance of grace—for her and me—and remembrance of my original goal of operating from my heart. This is a great model for life in general; it grows empathy and from there compassion flows. The adage of walking a mile in someone's shoes is another way of saying it, but, in the heat of a moment or hour, it requires stepping back and making space for the other's pain to dwell. The only pain I could feel at that point was my own.

Although I was doing all the suggested things like taking care of myself and spending early mornings in prayer and meditation, it wasn't helping. Life just sucked and was going to stay that way until I did something to change it. Mom had an expression when I was growing up. She was raising six kids, five of them boys, with a husband who was often absent. Whenever I heard this expression coming out of her mouth, I knew to give her space and quick. When she couldn't handle just one more thing, she'd declare in a loud voice, "I'm at my wits' end!" I was there. That's when the idea, unthinkable as it was, of moving Mom to an assisted living community was born.

Today's assisted living communities are a far cry from my grandmother's accommodations, but I was certain Mom's fear would prevail over anything remotely resembling one. A walker or wheelchair would set off a warning linked to memories and fears that lived deep in her psyche. I wasn't sure if she remembered those years with my grandmother, but I was sure she'd never lost her fear of nursing homes. Mom's untiring proclamation of, "I will not go to a nursing home," was permanently imbedded in my brain.

Assisted living facilities are not locked units. Fully comprehending Mom's determined nature, my greatest fear was that she would walk out. Not in search of someone like my grandmother but out of sheer resolve to go home. Mom didn't need a locked unit, but she did need moderate supervision, light help with bathing, healthy meals, assistance with medications, and daily social activities to keep her mind and body engaged.

Theoretically, if I removed Mom's fear of a nursing home, she would be the perfect candidate for assisted living because she loved people, staying busy, and going places. I would never have considered this scenario before, but I believed that sometimes life whittles us down to the point where we are forced to open our hands and let go of what we want, or think, the right thing is. That type of surrender opens doors to other possibilities, and, in my case, an option that I had been dead set against.

About this time, I started following a contemplative Franciscan priest, Father Richard Rohr, who, together with many other contemplative scholars including Thomas Merton, Cynthia Bourgeault, Henri Nouwen, and Thomas Keating eventually reshaped my understanding of religion, spirituality, and the way I live my life.

Fr. Richard believes that great love and great suffering are key experiences to transformation. In an excerpt from *Love and Suffering*, he writes, "Only love and suffering are strong enough to break down our usual ego defenses..."[40] This statement proved itself true in my walk with Mom during Alzheimer's, and time and time again as I confronted the suffering and sacrifices that go hand in hand with great love. I say great love because I've often loved, but it only became great when I pushed beyond what I—my preconceived notions, religion, or culture—thought was the acceptable depth, length, and bandwidth of love. Only after suffering myself, which almost always led to a shedding of thoughts, beliefs, and opinions that no longer served me, did I understand how love and suffering are so interconnected.

Fr. Richard goes on to say that if we love something enough, we will eventually suffer because of that love, and precisely because we've abandoned control to someone or something else. Everything we love will eventually change or come to an end in this life. Grief, in any form of loss—be it a physical loss of a loved one, a loss of hope, expectations, dreams, or the slow exit of an Alzheimer's loss—is, in my opinion, felt so deeply because we love so deeply.

Love and suffering, Fr. Richard believes, are universal human experiences, and "Without any doubt, they are the primary spiritual teachers more than any bible, church, minister, sacrament, or theologian."[41] I believe he is right because, despite what I have read, seen, or heard, nothing is quite as life-changing as walking through the fire and coming out the other side—banged up—yet somehow spiritually refined by the flames.

Alzheimer's was a firestorm of opportunities for testing the limits of love, and—strangely enough—understanding that the torment it caused in me created an opening that would eventually lead to somewhere better was helpful, especially toward the end of Mom's life when I navigated the most difficult days of the journey. For even if I didn't like where we were or think I could handle just one more thing, I kept the faith that this too would not only pass but pass into something that in time would reveal itself worthy of praise.

※ ※ ※

Mom was caught between the worlds of independence and dependence, and she hated the latter. Her memory was failing but not her need for autonomy. She was belligerent because everything she thought she wanted remained beyond the wall I was patrolling. Her cries to go home were really cries for independence, for the life she no longer had access to, for the life she would soon no longer remember.

Many things motivated me to consider assisted living and many things deterred me. I deliberated every scenario and outcome of moving Mom versus keeping her. My emotional state was like a flag on a windy day as my mind flipped back and forth: *keep her, move her, keep her, move her.* My physical exhaustion and mental torment begged for a decision, but, in the end, the thought of Mom recapturing a bit of the life stolen from her ultimately silenced my doubts and fears. That mindset gave rise to the possibility that things could be better there than they were here, that Mom just might be happy again, and that she would need to move to make that happen.

Chapter Twenty

It's All Coming Together

Summer 2010

*Once you make a decision, the universe
conspires to make it happen.*
Joseph Campbell

The excruciating decision to move Mom was behind us, but a more daunting task remained: how to get her there. When Mom didn't want to do something, she was a force no amount of cajoling, begging, or pleading could reckon with. Because of this, a lot of thought and planning went into devising a strategy that had the least potential for disruption and the most for success. The best chance for a win was also the path of least resistance. So, we lied to her.

During this time Mom had an ailing hip that was nearly bone to bone, and though even this failed to diminish her energy, the pain was flaring up. At eighty, her other hip had been replaced, and she'd recuperated in the rehab wing of a retirement community in Cincinnati. During that month-long process, she'd lived in a studio apartment and was able to access and enjoy all the amenities of independent living. She also had access to her sister and brother-in-law, who were full time residents there. She knew at the time it was a short-term stay, so the experience was pleasant for her.

My worst nightmare was Mom kicking and screaming all the way into assisted living, so I had to sell this just right. I had no idea how to pitch this whopper of a fib, but I remembered her good experience post-hip surgery, so I leveraged that. I explained that she needed to spend time rehabilitating her aching hip in a rehab wing of a retirement community. She was very wary at first, and I don't know if she even remembered her past stay. What she did know was that her hip was hurting, and, possibly because of that or divine intervention, she eventually, miraculously, agreed to the plan. At least I thought so.

We found Mom a studio apartment on the assisted living floor of a nearby community that accommodated independent living all the way through to memory care. When the day came to sign the paperwork, I was upfront in my request that Mom be able to age in place, and I was told that when the time came, with the assistance of hospice, most residents lived out their lives in memory care and didn't have to suffer another transition. It was a gentleman's agreement, not legally binding, and I chose to trust it.

Mom was moving to a beautiful, newer facility that boasted a busy daily activities schedule with lots of day trips, a walking fitness trail encompassing the property, plus an indoor pool. Her studio was small compared to what she was used to but beautifully decorated and easy to maneuver around.

I spent the weeks leading up to her move shopping and furnishing her room. During this time, she visited with my brother Mike and his family in Florida. My sister-in-law, Charlyne, flew in to help with the decorating. An excellent seamstress, she created an attractive duvet cover with matching window treatments and pillows for the bed and chairs. Mom's large picture window on the third floor overlooked the back parking lot to a landscaped area bordered by a swath of hardwoods and tall and graceful Georgia pines. Even in the winter those pines provided a green vista. She had a small kitchenette with cabinets and a countertop with a built-in microwave and mini refrigerator. There was even a comfortable sitting area with overstuffed chairs facing a credenza that held a large-screen TV. Some of her favorite keepsakes and family pictures adorned the tabletops and walls. It was warm, attractive, inviting, and so nice that the sales staff used her room as part of their tour to entice prospective residents and their families.

When the dubious moving day finally came, Mike and Charlyne (who was back home by that time) drove Mom from their home in St. Augustine directly to the assisted living wing of the retirement community. It was mid-afternoon when they arrived, and, as the three of them walked through the doors into the reception area, Mom was shocked but happy to see other family members there. Her sons and daughters-in-law had travelled from Cincinnati to meet my husband Steve and me to assist with the transition.

It was a celebratory atmosphere with lots of hugging and laughing, and Mom soaked it all up. She was in high spirits. A cynic by nature, she'd normally question everything surrounding this rehab stay. Not only had her family come from all over to see her, but her handsomely decorated studio had family pictures secured to the walls and familiar prized items placed throughout. Her wardrobe was hanging in the closet and folded in her drawers. We'd even stocked the kitchenette with plates and glasses, including her favorite snacks and refreshments.

Normally she'd have seen this ruse coming a mile away. But we were leaving her there, and she didn't have a clue. Physically she saw all the indicators of a long stay, but the communication bridge in her brain was down, blocking access to her natural skepticism. Alzheimer's was, as the gentleman in my support group had predicted, doing its part. Some of those neurons found ways to reestablish connection as the days trickled into weeks, and the weeks spilled into months, but, for that day, the plan was successful and all was well in Mom's transformed world.

We spent the afternoon touring the facility and enjoying wine in her room before she dressed for dinner. Mom picked out a pink pantsuit, her favorite color, as everyone in the community would soon come to know. She donned a white broad-brimmed floppy hat and wore stylish white gym shoes. She looked every inch the chic fashionista! Even in her mid-eighties she was striking with her thick, white mane and stunning blue eyes.

My brother Mike's memory fully captured the essence of Mom that evening as her high-spirited life force, missing over the past year, suddenly returned. He described a beautiful visual that still makes me smile, recalling her, "Skipping down the hall on the way to dinner!" She was surrounded by family, all dressed up, and eager to have dinner in a new restaurant. This was a good decision!

The glory of Mom was back!

Chapter Twenty-One

A New Life Is Born

Summer 2010

It takes love to hold on when you want to let go. It takes love to let go when you want to hold on.
Kate McGahan

The move had gone off without a hitch, but, days after, as the festivities ceased and my siblings returned home, Mom's cheerful state waned. Thinking I was helping her acclimate, I made the short drive every morning to arrive as she awakened and followed her around as she reluctantly joined the daytime activities. After lunch together, we'd walk the path around the beautiful grounds. I usually tried to leave before dinner, but it was hard because as I said goodbye, she'd beg to come home with me. This was ironic as just weeks earlier, she was begging to go home to Cincinnati.

The staff advised me to give her space to acclimate by herself. Every fiber in my body revolted against this guidance; it felt counterintuitive to completely disappear from a loved one thrust into an unknown environment and surrounded by total strangers. After doing research and talking to others, it looked to be mainstream advice, so I acted on it and gave her space—about fifty yards of it. Day after day I tucked my truck between other cars in the upper parking lot of assisted living, where I'd sit and watch the front door. She'd exit the building numerous times a day and stand under the portico, looking lonely, clutching her purse as she stared up the driveway. This breaking her in to her new home was also breaking my heart.

To an outside observer unaware of her disease, she held the stance of someone waiting for a bus or a friend to pick her up and whisk her away for a lunch date or an afternoon of shopping. She held that position for a good while before she turned around and went back inside. Then she'd resurface minutes later, and the cycle continued. At other times she came outside and sat by herself on the patio chairs. She spent a lot of time going in and out, and I spent a lot of time watching her.

I'd call the front desk, and they'd connect me to the director or the head nurse or whoever oversaw assisted living that day. I'd explain that Mom was spending a lot of time by herself again. They'd tell me she was strongly encouraged to participate in all the activities but not forced to do anything and that assisted living was a lot like independent living, but with added support. I knew they wanted her to acclimate as quickly as I did as they were extremely tired of my daily stalking and calling. They always ended the conversation by reminding me she'd eventually settle in.

I wasn't so sure about that. They didn't know my mom although, in trying to describe her determination, I threw out as many substitutes for unyielding as I could find. Peering through tear-stained eyes from the front seat of my truck, fully aware her mind couldn't comprehend the abandonment, I began to question all my motivations for moving her there. *What was I thinking? How could I have been so wrong? She needs to come back. But she can't come back. Where do I go from here?*

Weeks later, Mom still came outside to wait for the imaginary bus or friend but less frequently, and she began making real friends. I didn't hear that from her though when I called because she still complained about being there and repeatedly asked to go home, but her stance softened. The staff reported she was interacting with other residents and attending activities. As I observed from my hilltop perch, she was beginning to sit with a group of residents under the portico after dinner. I started to breathe again. Maybe this was had been the right decision after all.

When Mom and I spoke, she seemed to be adjusting, although somewhat unenthusiastically. She wasn't protesting as much to go home, so that was a win. She eventually regained a semblance of autonomy as she made decisions about her day, albeit small. She ran with a group of residents she called friends and did whatever they did.

What they did was attend one activity after another plus go on weekly outings. Slowly, she became part of a group that buzzed around the community like a beehive. The place kept the residents busy, and that worked for Mom. Her lapsed happiness was beginning to reappear, evident in her smile, her laughter, and her gait. She didn't forget me, as I was a constant in her life, but her new friends were becoming familiar. She was monitored by the staff, but at an unobtrusive distance so that she could still feel in control.

Eventually, Mom settled into a nice routine. I could join her for any of the meals, and the staff tried to match residents of similar cognitive levels during mealtimes, so the experience of eating became pleasurable for her again. Mary was her first mealmate and sat opposite her at the little table next to the window covered with white linen and fresh flowers. After breakfast, the two of them often walked the outside perimeter of the grounds. Every night at dinner she selected the following day's meals from a list of options. In the beginning she chose on her own, but toward the end of her stay she could no longer understand the concept of choices, and a staff member or I would choose for her.

There was a beauty salon in the building, where she had her hair done weekly, and a sweet aide did her nails in her room when we didn't go out for a manicure. Just like living independently, Mom could come and go as she chose with a friend or family member for the day or an extended period like a family vacation. Before long, I was seeing her daily and leaving freely although it took a couple of months to reach that point. Assisted living became her new home, and her new friends became her family. Mom had a new-fangled life. And so, in a way, did I.

Chapter Twenty-Two

Learning to Be Carried

Fall 2010

If you let go a little, you will have a little peace.
If you let go a lot, you will have a lot of peace.
            Ajahn Chah

Leaving mom in assisted living reminded me of leaving my boys on their first day of kindergarten—a painful parting for parent and child. Beginning their academic career was an exciting milestone on the road to independence, but it also launched the lifelong process of letting go. Andrea Matthews in an article titled "What Does It Mean to Let Go?" describes letting go as, "being willing to allow life to carry you to a new place, even a deeper, truer rendition of self. Holding on means trying to push life into the place of your liking or be damned."[42]

Alzheimer's is a master class on letting go—the ultimate release of everything we've known about a person in relationship to us. The heartbreaking reality is that while our loved ones may recognize us, and possibly remember our name, over time they may forget us as a daughter, son, wife, husband, partner, or friend. It's normal for people to forget us over the years as we move into different seasons of our lives, but we never dare dream it possible that we will lose all connection with those closest and most intimate to us, especially while they're still alive.

I had to let go of being someone's child even as an adult. Although I had just passed half a century on this earth and was a mother and grandmother myself, I was still a daughter in the eyes of someone else. Her safe harbor was a real place for me. Mom didn't just raise me; she also became my friend and confidante. And she was the family linchpin. How would forgetting her place in our world affect our family and our sibling dynamic?

Fortunately, releasing Mom from the role of a mom wasn't a disengagement from her because she still existed as the living and breathing individual who bore and raised me. Just because she didn't remember who she was, didn't mean I forgot who she was to me. Her lack of memory couldn't erase all the good and bad times, her years of love, sacrifice, laughter, and joy. What she had lost, I still stored and could recall. These experiences and memories still existed in me, and her laughter rang in my ears, but letting Mom go meant I needed to accept who she was, where she was, and that changed frequently. Our cadence altered, and I had to decide if we could still sway in the awful beauty of the Alzheimer's dance. I chose to dance, as I couldn't sit this one out, and the new moves required letting go of the old ones—the old Mom. I purposely grieved that part of her. We had an extraordinary mother-daughter relationship, but she was moving on, and I had to move with her. The only way to see and appreciate who she was at any given moment was to stop hanging on to who she used to be.

This was a hard-fought battle in my mind, and every time I chose to remain in the past—in that familiar place where Mom was still my mom, I recalled a memory: sitting in the kitchen of my childhood home, I was watching Mom as she argued with my grandmother. "Mother," Mom said in a frustrated voice, "that did not happen, you're making it all up." This was usually in respect to Ma's hysterically outlandish stories or confabulation as it is called. With a pained expression on her face, Mom was pleading with Ma to return to her, and Ma, a look of confusion in her eyes, had no idea what my mom was talking about. That memory was a teachable moment for me because holding on to my cherished memories of who Mom used to be was becoming more painful than letting her go and accepting who she had become. Somehow, the switch had been flipped, and I couldn't turn back.

So, who was Mom to me? She was the person who always had my back. No one in our lives cares about us quite the way a mother does. She worried too much and was convinced that I was not eating enough, not sleeping enough, or exercising too much. She told me truths the way only a mother could tell a daughter, using frank language like, "That color looks awful on you," or, "When's the last time you touched up your roots?" or, "I'm warning you, that friend is trouble." She loved my kids as her own, and, while a parent's love is usually enough, I realized that the benefits of unconditional love from another person with a long-range view of life are unparalleled. The things she told me that really didn't matter in life with respect to my kids, I came to find out, really didn't matter in the long run. Mom was direct, which could be annoying at times, but her love for family was as determined as her will was strong.

With Mom accepting her new life, I'd started to feel pretty good about my decision to move her. I thought she still knew me as a daughter, but I was preparing myself for the day when she didn't. I was well-read on dementia, and between Mom and Ma, was beginning to think I'd learned most of what Alzheimer's had to teach me. I should have known better.

I've heard it said that the worst experiences teach the best lessons because they deal directly with our five senses as opposed to forming ideas from others' encounters and insights. Learning from books and others can prepare us and often soften the blow of impending difficulties, but ultimately the experience is ours alone to taste, touch, smell, hear, and see. We absorb and remember it, good or bad, because we have walked it.

Mom was about half a year into her stay at assisted living when I stopped by one day between running errands. I spotted her immediately as I walked into the lobby. She was sitting with a group of residents waiting to board the bus for an afternoon outing. Mom looked up as I walked in, her eyes lighting up as she flashed me a big smile. Six months after her move, her cheerful greetings still filled me with unexpected joy as I never forgot the difficult months preceding and following her move. I had doubted she would ever be happy again.

As I approached, Mom stood up and exclaimed in a loud voice, "Oh look, my mother Marianne has come to visit." It was just a greeting, and most of the residents were used to seeing me with Mom, so no one seemed fazed by her comment. Some of the residents were there because of physical challenges but most were equally as confused as Mom. I was the only one who caught the mistake, which I brushed off, saying hello to the group and making small talk until the bus came. I walked out with the chatty little cluster, watching as the driver assisted everyone aboard. Mom waved to me from the window as the bus pulled out. I continued to wave back until the bus turned the corner at the top of the hill.

I remained in that position under the portico for a while, eyes locked on the last sighting of the little white bus with blue letters splashed across its side. I guess I hoped it would reappear, reverse down the hill, and park back under the portico. Then the residents would file out of the bus and into the lobby where they were seated before I arrived. I would walk in, and Mom would greet me, introducing me as Marianne, her daughter.

Just as the bus disappeared from my sight that day, so did my identity as a daughter. And not only that, but Mom's lapse also wiped out the generations after me: my kids and grandkids. If she didn't know me, she didn't know them. Words can't fully describe the feeling but "left behind" came close. Although I could still try to meet Mom wherever she was in her journey, it would no longer be as a daughter—every trace of that relationship had just vanished, and in that void an unfamiliar loneliness crept in.

There is no good preparation for this type of loss—all my research, listening to others, and convincing myself I was doing the right thing couldn't come close to the day when Mom was no longer my mom. I was married to my college sweetheart, the love of my life, with three amazing sons, a sweet granddaughter, a big extended family, and close friends. My life was good, but I knew then there would always be a hole in me that only one person could fill.

Mother was one of many titles I assumed, but I was always someone Marianne. When I wasn't her mother, I was her *friend* Marianne. The following week I was her *sister* Marianne, *cousin* Marianne, or *Aunt* Marianne. Losing her this way brought on an ache that came in waves—initially a shock to my system, but eventually it became easier. Over time it brought me to the place where I started having fun with my many titles, laughing with Mom about our adventures as sisters or friends. What else was there to do but go with the flow?

No matter what she called me, I could still feel her love and that became enough. It had to be. "Enough," according to an old Buddhist proverb, "is a feast." I just had to let go, a lot, which equaled a feast of peace, and there in that bountiful banquet of acceptance, life was beginning to carry me.

Chapter Twenty-Three

Apprehended by Awe

Fall 2010

*He to whom the emotion is a stranger, who can no longer
pause to wonder and stand wrapped in awe,
is as good as dead; his eyes are closed.*
Albert Einstein

Most individuals experience wonder and awe as a physical phenomenon. They feel the warm water lapping at their toes and the sun kissing their face before they see that enormous ball of hydrogen and helium light up the sky in a grand finale of yellows and oranges just before fading. Sometimes it's the soothing effect of a musical piece that lifts them out of the present moment and allows their soul to soar before returning. Awe is those moments of ethereal pauses from the ordinary that let us know there is something extraordinary before us.

Perhaps my expectations of Mom's move were so low that when everything fell into place and I saw her happiness return, I entered a sustained state of wonder. That was partly true as my hopes were cautious, to say the least, but I think there was more to it. Maybe awe just happens in those moments of allowing, when we remain open and blank to what's unfolding right in front of us without commentary or the need to analyze, influence, or judge.

During this period of grace as I like to call it or this surprising chapter in Mom's life, she was really having fun. I would compare those years to summer camp. Her activities director was the camp counselor who created and attended the many functions. Mom's little cluster of friends flitted from one activity to another, all day long, so they never got bored. After a full day, three meals, and two snacks, she was content, and she slept well at night. She had aides who assisted with showering, and nurses to distribute medication. Her room was cleaned daily, her laundry done weekly.

There were parallels to managing Mom's Alzheimer's and raising my boys. When my sons were small, I kept them active with mental and physical activities. They were rarely bored and consistently got good sleep. Like my sons, Mom thrived when she was engaged. That could be as simple as singing favorite oldies around a piano with others or as complex as an easy jigsaw puzzle. Activities that required complex thought or planning frustrated her, but she could follow simple, straightforward directions.

Much like my grandmother, Mom loved to talk on the phone. She never owned a cell phone, so she used the land line in her studio. She was highly responsive to calls from family members and friends, which happened daily and usually in the early mornings. Sometimes I'd call and get a busy signal for hours. Concerned she was becoming the teenager who stayed on the phone, I'd call the nurses' station to check on her. They'd look in her room, find it empty, and eventually find her with a group of residents somewhere in the building. What we came to discover was that at some point during a phone conversation, she just dropped the receiver on the bed and hurried out the door, forgetting to hang up.

Every day in assisted living was different. After breakfast Mom usually went for a walk and then off to her first activity. That might be outside potting plants, tai chi, or a group nature walk then back inside for lunch. The afternoon offered manicures, arts and crafts, musical entertainers, shuffleboard, or cookie decorating. Pet therapy was also on the menu, and, of course, she had her own pet therapy whenever I brought Abby, who now lived with me. There were many outings to museums, movies, local playhouses, and lunch establishments that Mom never missed. Dinners in the independent dining room created occasions for Mom to dress up and feel like she was going somewhere special. After we were seated, she often commented, "I just love this little restaurant." Dinner was often followed by movie nights, bible reading, old time radio hour, or unstructured leisure time. On nice evenings, Mom and her new group of friends often went outside and sat under the portico.

Mom and I also enjoyed doing things outside of the structured activities. On pleasant afternoons, we'd often walk to the independent living side of the retirement community, grab an ice cream from the cooler at the small market, and head outside to the covered porch overlooking the woods. We lost hours swaying back and forth in those oversized rockers while enjoying our creamy treats. Sometimes Mom asked to pray the rosary, and sometimes she fell asleep rocking.

I saw Mom at some point every day, sometimes joining her for activities, sometimes just popping in to say hi. Often, we went out for lunch or dinner, shopping, or to a movie. It dawned on me one day that I was having fun with Mom, and she was enjoying me too. I became one of those lovely ladies I'd hired while mom had been living with me. After so many years of frustration and angst, dating to her diagnosis of MCI in Ohio, we were so good that I didn't constantly dwell on what was going on in her brain. It didn't matter that our relationship had changed or that I was introduced as her aunt, or sister, or whoever—we were back to doing all the fun things mothers and daughters do. Even if our roles were reversed or all mixed up, the love remained. I was in awe!

CHAPTER TWENTY-FOUR

Saved by Friendship

2010 Onward

*I would rather walk with a friend in the dark,
than alone in the light.*
HELEN KELLER

Assisted living occupants were all ages with different stories and unique mental or physical disabilities. There were residents there for purely physical reasons, but they followed the same schedule of assisted living activities as the cognitively challenged, and most, but not all, mingled right beside their confused friends.

It was a good mix for Mom as she talked to anybody who would listen, and those without neurological dysfunction mentally stimulated her. As I watched Mom and her co-inhabitants interact, I observed that despite the differences in mental abilities, they all had one thing in common. Their obvious desire for companionship. Well beyond their disorders, an inherent need for human interaction persisted.

The cognitively challenged didn't know each other's names or pasts, and no one knew or cared about previous positions and titles previously held. Who you had been didn't matter, because all you had was who you were now. They became one in their human brokenness, buzzing around the building in search of their next adventure.

Mom loved this communal environment, but hands down the biggest reasons she acquiesced to her move and adjusted so well were two individuals she bonded with in ways I never thought possible after Alzheimer's. Social connections had always been at the core of her personality; she maintained many lifelong friendships dating from grade school, but after she got sick even these relationships watered down to superficial states. I was sure she had lost the ability to develop authentic connections and learn new things, but I sure was wrong. She mastered and remembered her way around the entire retirement community as well as the outside grounds. Although she forgot the names of those family members and friends not seen on a regular basis, she remembered me and those two other special individuals: Lucy and Morrie.

It wasn't just that she remembered their names, she also developed meaningful relationships with them. Going beyond superficial friendship requires skills like thoughtfulness and sensitivity—traits I hadn't seen in Mom since sometime after her diagnosis. Her ability to establish and continue these bonds was an indication of more going on in Mom than I gave credit for, and I wondered why that was.

What part did stress play in Mom's behaviors when she was living with me, and did it also play a partial role in her developing dementia in the first place? Not that stress was avoidable after Alzheimer's because most of it was fueled by her yearning for her long-term memories—like her home—and her inability to connect with her short-term memories. Stress releases cortisol into the blood stream, which is necessary in fight or flight situations. However, prolonged exposure to this hormone, among other things, is known to halt the production of new brain cells and fracture the connections between the neurons, which in turn causes the cells to die and the brain to shrink. All these factors not only affect the brain's ability to remember the pot of carrots left on the burner, a familiar route, or a son's name but also its ability to store and process information that is essential to living.

Perhaps Mom's lack of stress at this point in her journey cleared the fog in her mind a bit, allowing her to recover some of the life that was taken from her. I was pleased at her progress but also blown away when occasionally I'd show up and Mom would greet me then turn right around and continue with her friends. It reminded me of picking my grandkids up at daycare and them asking for just five more minutes. Seriously? They didn't want to stay there in the morning but didn't want to leave their friends in the afternoon! I didn't mind this at all though because it revealed an emotional state that allowed Mom to feel safe and secure in her new space and with her new family. Just knowing that freed up my mind and my schedule!

Mom's social connections undeniably improved her cognition as well as her sense of well-being. Her mind was less conflicted—most likely the result of losing most of her Cincinnati memories. Just as I'd been told, Alzheimer's was giving her brain a break. Forgetting her past allowed her to live fully in the present, where she once again enjoyed the benefits and beauty of friendship!

Her first friend was Morrie, and everyone comes across someone like him in their lifetime. He's that well-groomed, extremely social guy who enjoys working the crowd and is always ready with a story or joke. He makes it a point to remember everyone's name, and a compliment is usually the first thing off his tongue. People like Morrie are always smiling and never seem to have a bad day.

The Morrie we came to know and love didn't remember everyone's name, but he still greeted everyone with a smile, and a "Hey fella" to any of the men in his path. He moved from independent to assisted living shortly before Mom arrived. Morrie charmed our whole family, and we thoroughly enjoyed interacting with him.

Like most men in his generation, he'd served in the military and was passionate about his service. He readily repeated stories of his Navy gunner days and his travels around the world. Morrie's wife passed shortly before he moved to assisted living, but his eyes lit up as he recalled her and their life together. Slowly flipping through pictures in his wallet, his eyes glistened as he caressed the old, worn photos while recalling their beautiful waltzes together. She was an artist, and as he described her pieces, he was simultaneously pulling you to his studio where many of her paintings adorned the walls.

Morrie was fun-loving and playful with Mom, but always in a proper way. She was a sponge, soaking up all the attention he lavished on her. They spent a lot of time within the confines of the larger group, always sitting next to each other during activities and events. They were equally high-spirited, both loving to laugh and sing and dance.

There were occasions when Mom and Morrie landed in her room after their group disbanded for the evening, sitting in front of her TV sipping a beer or glass of wine. Although she liked the occasional cocktail when family visited, they were mostly for that reason. But these two enjoying a drink alone raised some serious eyebrows with the staff, so I quickly cleaned out any remaining alcohol.

There were numerous themed events and dinners held in the independent section of the community open to assisted residents and their families. Mom attended every one. She'd pick an outfit with a matching hat, and I would curl her hair and apply make-up. Her face would beam like a birthday girl in anticipation of her party as we excitedly made our way to the other side of the building. She loved any excuse to dance. I remember Kevin and Cathy once travelled from Cincinnati to attend a Monte Carlo event. After we made our way through the casino games, Mom spotted the dance floor and was quick to cut a rug. She danced the traditional slower songs with my husband, brother, and, of course, Morrie. Then she kicked it up a notch as the tempo picked up and she bopped to the fox trot and twirled to the tango. Morrie was always right alongside her; the two of them were the community's own Fred Astaire and Ginger Rogers. She would have shut down another dance floor that night had it not been for the fall. As country music blared through the speakers, she two-stepped it right off the custom-built platform. Luckily it was only a slight drop, and she escaped with minor injuries.

Morrie and Mom fed off each other's high level of energy. He was Doctor Fun to her, and she lit up any time she saw him, but there was another, much more intimate relationship that blossomed with Mom, and that friendship continued into memory care.

Lucy was slightly slumped over, but steady on her feet and always held her head high as she slowly made her way forward in her walker. Her white-gray hair was usually salon styled, and although heavily lined, I never saw her face devoid of a warm and inviting smile. She embodied the contentment of one at peace with her life, even as she was surrounded by individuals at lesser cognitive levels.

She was already in assisted living when Mom moved in, and the two of them quickly became late-life soulmates. If Morrie was sitting on one side of Mom, Lucy was on the other. Morrie appealed to Mom's sense of excitement and adventure, but Lucy was quiet and doting, and Mom grew to love her deeply. Lucy had served as a nurse in the Navy during WWII, and her peaceful and caring manner had a calming effect on Mom. Their relationship was sweet and affectionate, and it was evident to everyone who witnessed them.

Mom had several lifelong friendships. These were with cousins and friends who became sisters and confidants—and people we considered family growing up. Bernice was one of those friends Mom met in grade-school, and she possessed many of the same attributes as Lucy. I often wondered how Mom and Lucy could became so close so late in life, and especially considering Mom's dementia, but I believe that Lucy represented Bernice to Mom on some level, not in appearance, but certainly in demeanor.

Mom and Lucy didn't always talk, and while they sometimes carried on about things, they mostly seemed content just being in each other's company. They would take their afternoon snack to Mom's room and sit at her café table, chatting away as they consumed their treats. They looked out for each other, like an old married couple, each of whom feels incomplete without the other.

I have a touching memory that I often replay in my mind. Steve and I were walking behind them one evening as they made their way down the hall in the direction of their studios. Lucy was holding on to her walker, which was slightly in front of her, and Mom was beside her. They began to sing, and as they did their bodies swayed in gentle rhythm from side to side. Their voices crooned out an old song remembered from days past, and they continued in that unhurried dance all the way to Lucy's room.

Like teenage girls, they had sleepovers. I didn't know this until one evening as I was helping Mom prepare for bed. She was in the bathroom, and I was watching TV when there was a knock at the door. Before I could get up Lucy entered, barefoot and clad in her nightgown. She had come to let Mom know that her couch was ready with a sheet, blanket, and a pillow. She said her door was unlocked, and told Mom she could come whenever she was ready. Sure enough, as I walked Mom to Lucy's room on my way out, the couch was set up just as she'd said with a blanket neatly folded over the sheet. The only thing missing was popcorn and a movie for these sweet sisters to complete their slumber party!

Angels do walk amongst us, and I would be remiss if I didn't mention another individual who moved in during the latter part of Mom's stay in assisted living. This was Sam, and he was an exceptionally tenderhearted gentleman who was considerably younger, wheelchair bound, and completely cognizant. Surrounded by individuals with varying degrees of mental decline, he was stuck in their sphere of confusion, but it wasn't apparent by the way he interacted with them.

Sam was a gift, especially to Mom, but also to many others. He could look beyond the mental fog of the residents and find a way to connect with them, which can be difficult with individuals suffering from dementia. I didn't know his entire story, but I do believe hardship renders humility. His resilient and cheerful attitude intrigued me, and I often found myself watching him as he meandered about the building. He wasn't a teacher, but I learned so much by witnessing his generous and compassionate heart.

Smiling enthusiastically, he'd roll up to another resident and lavish them with an encouraging affirmation. His sincerity was palpable, and I saw firsthand how he could quickly transform a gloomy face into a bright smile. He seemed to seek out the lonely. After lunch he'd often be found in his wheelchair out on the sidewalk taking in the late afternoon sun. Spying us as we walked the fitness path, he'd holler out to Mom, "Hi Pat, how is your day going?" or, "Pat, you sure do look pretty in pink."

That's all it took. Mom would immediately alter our course and talk to him. She never remembered his name, but her face would beam whenever she saw him. There wasn't much reciprocal conversation as Mom did all the talking, repeating the same stories over and over, but Sam listened, ever so patiently. His eyes rested on hers as he leaned forward, smiling and nodding as if she was the most important person on the planet. He gave the occasional and well placed, "Wow," or, "That's great," and always ended the conversation with a handshake or high five. That made her day, and he seemed to gain immense pleasure from seeing her smile.

As I reflect on this period of Mom's journey, I am still blown away by these memories. Considering our tragic family history with this disease and the fairly predictable timeline of mental decline with Alzheimer's, I had hoped for some semblance of a life for her, but I'd never expected what transpired. I knew this phase was short-lived in the grand scheme of Alzheimer's—the next shoe was going to drop. But this time I hoped to avoid the anticipatory anxiety that accompanies that presumption—as true as it might be—by simply enjoying Mom as she delighted in her new life for as long as that lasted. She was happy and having fun—what more could I, and Mom, have asked for?

All the individuals at Mom's facility had stumbled into some type of darkness that changed the trajectory of their lives, ending up in a place where no one wants to go and surrounded by strangers. Their response to this new world was an inherent reaction imprinted on their souls since birth; they reached out to one another. It didn't require a healthy mind or a functional body, only an indwelling need for love. They embraced each other and were saved by friendship!

Chapter Twenty-Five

Patty Re-Invented

2010 Onward

Toto, I have a feeling we're not in Kansas anymore.
L. Frank Baum

Mom wasn't anywhere anymore that she remembered, but it didn't hold her back. Those precious borrowed days in assisted living brought back memories of letters received from my son, Ryan, while at summer camp. His notes were short but always spoke of new friends and depicted exciting adventures. Originally, I didn't think he'd survive, much less flourish, away from home, but left to his own accord he discovered his inner force. It took Mom many years after her diagnosis, mostly due to her internal unrest, but eventually she rediscovered hers.

When her spirited force broke through the barriers of Alzheimer's, a new chapter was written introducing a whole new cast. The leading characters were Morrie, Sam, and Lucy. As they stepped onto the stage of *Patty's Story*, the overhead lights cycled brilliant hues of red, blue, orange, yellow, and, of course, pink. They colored Mom's world with love, laughter, and fun. She found a life, and I found her. She recognized me, but not as her daughter. I recognized her, but not as my mom.

She didn't have old memories, but she still had a life and that begged the question, does remembering who we were before Alzheimer's make us who we really are? In *The Grapes of Wrath*, the men and women burned or sold their possessions because those things represented a past that had been destroyed. They then wondered how they could live their lives without the stuff that symbolized their past.

Could Mom know who she was without her stuff—not her physical stuff but her memories of the roles she played and the people in them? If our life is only our memories, then the inability to recall them would not only strip us of our humanity but also the vital part of us that travels beyond this earthly existence. Mom's lack of memory took her identity as a mother as well as the other titles she was called. At times it took her ability to reason and be reasonable, and over time it took her ability to communicate. Ultimately it took her life. But it never took her soul.

She didn't remember her past, but I witnessed firsthand her strong-willed soul reinvent her life with the same hunger and zeal displayed before Alzheimer's. That revealed, at least to me, she was still in there and determined to be seen and heard in whatever form that took—and it took many. Despite her being my friend, cousin, aunt, or even thinking I was her mother, her feisty nature and deeply rooted attributes remained.

That's who I came to meet every morning—her life force—and it's within all of us however we define it. Sometimes it's deeply buried under all the labels that we, and the world, project on us. These descriptions have us believe we are only as real or valuable as our physical prowess, our status in life, and our mental aptitude and cognizance. But who we are at the deepest level of our being is where we connect with God. Alzheimer's couldn't touch that, and as Mom's cousin Jim used to say, referring to Mom's strong spirit, "When God made Patty, He threw away the mold!" He knew there was no one quite like Mom, and she couldn't be silenced!

Ironically, this thief had a silver lining, for as it slipped out the back with the goods, it also snatched distractions most of us encounter daily: worry and anxiety about the future, regrets from the past, material wants, and the need for fame or power. The more Mom forgot that stuff, the freer she became to live the life that unfolded right in front of her. Amazingly, she was able to attain a state of mind most of us struggle a lifetime to achieve; she was living in the moment, and in those moments, she rediscovered her life.

Although detached from her original narrative in life, she was no less significant or valuable. She was just Patty, a name given to her at birth that no longer signified any definite role. Despite that, she was still a social butterfly fluttering around her new world. She maintained her love of clothing and sense of fashion, styled her beautiful mane, and applied her makeup every morning—pink was still her favorite color, always adorning her lips. She continued to love music, dancing, parties, and outings. Just like the old days, there were people she was naturally drawn to and people she didn't care for. There was one ill-tempered, snappy resident who really got under Mom's skin, and she scared the heck out of me. Whenever we would see her, Mom would lean in close and whisper, in a not-so-quiet voice, "There's the pill."

Before Alzheimer's robbed Mom of her ability to remember so many things, not the least of which was who she was to me, I would have surely cringed at this remark, closing my eyes, and praying the intended target of Mom's words didn't hear them. But as obnoxious as it was, it made me pretty happy. We'd come a long way, Mom and I, and I could finally see that despite all the loss, she was still the same spunky soul I always knew and loved—defects and all!

Her sparkle returned as she loved, laughed, and danced her way through another life on this earth. An ember shorter in duration but still as hot and bright as the original fire. She wasn't in Kansas anymore, but Patty was not yet ready to hang up her dance shoes.

Chapter Twenty-Six

Fighting the Establishment

Late 2012

If you want a happy ending, that depends, of course, on where you stop your story.
Orson Welles

If this was fiction, my story could end here. I would tell how Mom lived happily ever after in this confused but mostly happy state until she passed peacefully in her sleep. For me, it would have been enough—a feast—to know her colorful soul existed beyond her brain damage, but there was more to come. Assisted living was the last dance before her ballet slippers wore down. And as the curtain began falling on that remarkable scene, I wasn't blind to what lay behind; I had been given the unmistakable gift of sight.

To an outsider she was diminished, and in truth she was. She may not have known the day, understood her relationships or why she lived where she lived, but she lived, and she lived with passion. Recognizing Mom beyond a mother was more than I could have ever asked for, even though that wasn't the answer I sought early on in this journey. But through the process of *trying* to recognize her, a pivotal moment in my faith emerged.

Like many others, I've prayed, for situations, for people, and for outcomes. Sometimes, those prayers have been answered although not usually on my timetable. My dealings with God, up to this point, were more of a transactional nature—give and take, mostly take, and, "I promise to do this if You promise to do that." To many it may seem like a rudimentary concept, but I finally understood that in the sheer act of asking God to show me Mom through her dementia, I was already receiving. The flow of grace had begun in the asking, allowing the blinders to work themselves loose. I would have never asked if I didn't already believe, even in my uncertainty, that it was possible. Acquiring that vision of Mom began with the faith to ask for it.

Mom was slowing down, but still doing well within the expected parameters for assisted living. As with an engaging book that captures the heart, I never wanted that chapter in her story to end because I knew what would follow. I couldn't have imagined anything better than the gift I'd already received, but there was more to come. I just had to swim through some rough waters first.

I received an odd meeting request from the assisted living director. She didn't share any details, and I had no reason to suspect anything other than the quarterly progress report. That assumption changed when I walked into her office and saw she was joined by two other administrative staff members. They smiled as I entered, but the air held a tension. My heart sank as I observed them seated around the table with hands folded on top of files. I slowly lowered myself into the chair, sensing something unpleasant was about to unfold.

After exchanging greetings, they dove right in and told me they were concerned Mom had progressed to the point where she needed "more specialized care." They said she was requiring "more help" getting ready in the mornings, and evenings. They were worried she might become a "flight risk" although she never wandered off. They didn't offer the solution many others in assisted living utilized when they needed more help, which was part-time paid aides. They gave no concrete reasons to move her, other than to say, "In our opinion, it's time."

I was confused and asked them to repeat what they were asking of me. I questioned whether they had the right patient file. It wasn't a joke; they knew who Mom was, but I was so shocked and blindsided that I needed to double check. Although there was decline in some areas, there were no indications Mom was struggling with this level of care, no dialogue, no forewarnings from any of the staff who dealt directly with her.

I could have understood if I'd just been a Sunday visitor, or even a daily call-in, totally unaware of Mom's status, but I saw her most every day. I knew her condition better than anyone. I was that helicopter daughter who made it a point to know and communicate with all the staff involved with Mom, from Susan the receptionist at the front desk Mom passed on her daily walk to the maids who tidied up her room and everyone in between. I did not see the depths of decline they were describing. There's no escaping the progressive pathway of Alzheimer's, but I knew she wasn't ready for a locked unit. I also knew that a drastic change in her environment could easily traumatize her and send her spiraling—just like Ma.

My mind raced to consider other possibilities. Perhaps a couple of the independent residents had complained? When Mom couldn't walk outside, she made her way from assisted to and the independent side of the building and back. Because of that a lot of the residents on her route knew her, and knew she had dementia. Since I often walked with her, I knew she'd stop, say hello, and make small talk to everyone she passed or at least try. Most seemed happy to see her and were sweet, but I did occasionally catch a snarky reaction. I assumed people thought Alzheimer's was contagious and didn't want to get anywhere near her. I understood that. For them, Mom was the grim reminder of an unpreventable disease that dramatically increases with age, especially past eighty.

I also wondered if Mom's cane had led to this meeting. She did have incidents that called for conversations with the staff because occasionally that cane took on a life of its own as it banged against slow elevator doors. I had spoken with her about this, but she was just like my grandmother when the ice cream went missing—deny, deny, deny. Of course, it was also pointless having that conversation because she couldn't remember doing anything with the cane before the conversation, and, for the same reason, didn't remember after.

I understood my viewpoint was somewhat subjective because I wasn't with Mom 24/7. But outside of the cane incidents, which to my knowledge only happened a few times, I saw no beneficial reason to move her. She blended well within a group and was especially close to a couple of individuals. She attended all the social activities and was happy, albeit confused. On her daily walks inside and outside of the building, she never got lost or failed to return.

Despite this, the meeting I was asked to attend was not actually a conversation—it was a lecture. There was no exchange of anything, just information and opinions being doled out on one side and received on the other. I was being served by three well-prepared administrative staff members whose goal was to move Mom upstairs, to memory care, whether she was cognitively ready or not. During my frequent conversations with shift nurses and aides who worked directly with Mom, no one ever alluded to these concerns. In speaking to the same individuals after the meeting, not one of them agreed with the administrators' assessment.

My lack of preparation for this discussion was evident in my lack of response and dumbfounded expression as my eyes moved from person to person. Overwhelmed, my brain drew a blank. I felt heat rising in my face and my heart trying to pound its way out of my ribs; I understood its anxiety because I wanted out too. After a while they indicated the meeting was over by offering to take me upstairs and tour memory care. Dazed, I nodded at their suggestion and followed them to the elevator.

I was frightened for Mom; her greatest fear was a locked unit. My heart continued to race as we entered the elevator. No one said a word. The slow rise from floor to floor matched my emotions as the initial shock and befuddlement escalated to a higher pitch—anger. I'd been pummeled by a blow I didn't see coming. Their triple-layered offensive strategy kept me off guard. I struggled to keep my emotions in check as I stared down at the elevator floor, but I also began to recover and thought about my options. Could I move Mom into another community at this point? Yes. Would it have been in her best interest? No. Assisted living creates a culture of consistency and predictability for dementia residents. Moving Mom would be a stressor to her system that would surely plunge her deeper into Alzheimer's. It would be cruel.

We exited the elevator onto the fourth floor and into a small hallway. In Mom's time in assisted living, I'd never ventured near this floor although I knew it was there. I just wouldn't let my mind go to that eventuality if she was still thriving where she was. Assisted living had been a huge step and one that had turned out better than I'd hoped, but a locked unit was an entirely different ball game. Memory care, as far as I was concerned, was on the other side of the planet.

Someone punched a code in the keypad to access the unit. There it was, that small rectangular box on the wall programmed with a series of numbers that allowed access on one side while denying it on the other. Soon enough the day would come when I would input a sequence of numbers to access Mom, but not then. She was still too cognitively aware of her surroundings and friends, too physically and socially active, and too mindful of her independence. It didn't make sense that they wanted to move her, and neither she nor I was in any way ready for it.

Like water boiling in a pot, these thoughts bubbled in my brain. I was cynical and didn't trust the system. I considered the very real possibility they were trying to make a room available for someone in independent living needing more help because the assisted living studios were full. Aging in place is a philosophy that implies the resident can live out their life in one community, and when they need more help, there will be a room available at the higher skill level. But what happens when there's not a vacancy?

The administration left me with the nurse in charge of memory care to lead the tour. I listened respectfully as she described a day in the life of a memory care resident. I took in all the sweet souls sitting in the living area, some watching me as I watched them. Many of those same individuals would eventually become family to me. On this day, though, I had to become Mom's voice and stand up for what I knew to be true. She was not ready for this, and I would not hasten her downward spiral a single day by allowing it.

The tour ended, and I left the unit. Composing myself in the hallway on the other side of the locked door, I dried my tears with my sleeve and rode the elevator down to the first floor. I deliberated everything said in the meeting and gained a foot of confidence for every inch that painstakingly slow elevator descended. As the doors opened, I walked through the common area into the director's office, closing the door behind me. When I reemerged sometime later, it was completely understood and undeniably clear that Mom was not going to memory care, not on that day.

I made the necessary adjustments to ensure that Mom was not requiring more assistance than anyone else. I arrived early in the mornings to help her shower and dress and hired aides to assist her nightly bedtime ritual. She was completely capable of handling her day in between. I didn't know how long Mom would remain in assisted living, but even one day outside of a locked unit was well worth the fight. For Mom, it was six months, one hundred and eighty days to be with her sweet family, while allowing her spirit to roam free before it was forever curbed.

This sweet chapter in Mom's journey did end, not unexpectedly, but still sadly. Life is full of both happy and unhappy endings, all bearing unique gifts that impart wisdom when the time is right. These ephemeral seasons weave in and out of our lives, and I've found that if I don't like the current ending, I must be patient and hang on through the storm, because, just like the weather in the south, it will give way to a new one. And it did.

Chapter Twenty-Seven

Moving Upstairs

2013

The world is quiet here.
Lemony Snicket

Like clockwork, the administration circled around with another assessment around the six-month mark. This time there was a consensus of opinion, including mine although still with some reservations, that Mom was ready to move upstairs. I may never have been completely sure, and I realized that, but I was better prepared, and I believed Mom's memory had diminished to the point where she wouldn't struggle. Of course, she kept surprising me!

For the first few weeks in memory care, when Mom was up and dressed, she would make her way toward the common area in her walker, purse in tow. Then, instead of sitting down for breakfast, she would bypass the tables and bolt for the exit as fast as her legs could push. Arriving there, she furiously attempted to turn the handle, and, when that didn't work, she dealt that door a rapid succession of blows with her fists. The staff were sometimes able to distract her with breakfast, but shortly after she was at it again. Her battle cry to go home returned, but this time she yearned for the freedom of the floor below, and the camaraderie of her late-life companions, especially Lucy.

Mom's studio room in memory care was exactly one floor up from her old room, a bit smaller in square footage, and without the kitchenette. Everything else, including the view from her window, the positioning of the furniture, window treatments, and pictures on the wall were the same. She was comfortable and content within the confines of that familiar environment, but all that changed when she left her room and entered the common area where the memory care residents spent most of their days.

Mom was no different from the residents unaffected by Alzheimer's in that she tried to keep up with those at a higher level. Their mental acuity motivated hers. I was on board with moving Mom, but I was concerned how the difference in cognitive levels she would encounter in memory care would affect her, and I was very worried about her leaving Lucy. Her cognition was toward the higher end of memory care, as opposed to being at the lower end when she left assisted living, so I braced for a significant decline.

Even in her limited capacity, Mom tried consistently to communicate with others. She often got smiles and nods, but not much conversing back and forth. I saw this happening but conceded. Perhaps it was a rationalization that helped me feel better, but I accepted the realization that this was the season where Mom could finally stop trying so hard. Her tenacious soul could finally take pause from bellowing out to be seen and heard. And unlike the woman who had constantly needed something to do every minute of the day, she seemed at ease with being at ease.

This place wasn't my grandmother's first nursing home, which I regarded as a waiting room for the dying. There was a quiet worthiness to these individuals and a dignity in the approach to their care from the head nurse to the aides and the housekeepers. This was most evident though in the activities director, who was able to connect and work with everyone, individually and collectively. It was quite an accomplishment considering the many different cognitive stages of her charges.

Mom and the others upstairs were confined to a common area where dining, morning stretches, art activities, and balloon volleyball took place. Entertainment and dog therapy came to them. Memory care felt like an intimate family unit that operated quietly together as opposed to the smaller but more energetic groups in assisted living. This appeared to work well for residents in the final phase of their journeys.

Despite considerable decline in the last six months of assisted living, Mom still fought for the freedom beyond the door and the faces she loved below. Meanwhile, according to Lucy's family, she was equally miserable downstairs in assisted living. A few months after Mom's move, Lucy's family made the decision to move her into memory care, and the duo was back together. Mom's agitation abated with Lucy by her side, and she eased into a nice routine. They were once again inseparable and often found in each other's rooms just sitting quietly. I sensed an ancient familiarity between them, one often reserved for individuals who had spent a lifetime together.

The residents were rounded up daily and led in some type of activity or group exercise. Mom and I still walked the outside grounds, at first with her walker and later in a wheelchair. The enclosed outdoor patio area, which was only accessed by a code, was one of her favorite places to sit on pretty days and listen to music or move her fingers slowly along the beads as I prayed the rosary.

Some of the nurses' aides were extraordinarily kind, giving her manicures, curling her hair, and applying makeup. She loved that. In the evenings after she was dressed for bed, one aide often sat with her as she fell asleep. She ate and slept well, an indicator of overall peace of mind. Her biggest angst came whenever we left the building for a doctor's appointment as memory care had become her new security blanket.

The overall busyness of Mom's life in assisted living decelerated in memory care. It was a slower dance with a unique soothing rhythm. Equanimity was more apparent within those walls, despite housing courageous souls who fiercely campaigned in the battlefield of the brain. Their work was near completion, and at times I could almost hear a collective sigh and sense their soul's readiness as freedom waited patiently in the wings.

They still had much to say, not literally in most cases, but by their smiles and laughter, outbursts, and sometimes in their tears. The moments of compassion and tenderness I saw in those individuals considered severely demented overwhelmed me. "How could such goodness coexist with such hopelessness," I often wondered. Little acts are sometimes lacking within a healthy cognitive population but were often visible in that small unique universe tucked away from the rest of society. Their acts of kindness may have been slight, but they spoke volumes about the heart behind the outwardly absent individual.

Many times, I witnessed a gentleman get up from the couch to let Mom or another female sit down in his place, and other times someone would pick up the dropped baby doll, tenderly re-wrap the blanket around it, and place it back in the lap of the woman who always sat in the rocker cradling her swaddled bundle. There was another woman in residence who randomly cried, and although she always got stares her way, there was one sweet lady who would slowly push her way out of her chair, cross the room, and sit next to her and hold her hand.

Not to say there weren't occasional flare-ups. These were still people with individual likes, dislikes, and feelings, and sometimes these presented in anger—different from the outbursts I commonly saw in the earlier stages of Alzheimer's with Mom's inability to communicate effectively or her outrage at not being able to go home. What I noticed in memory care was more typical of individuals who sometimes get on each other's nerves because they live together, such as impatience because one of them is not moving fast enough or another stands in front of the TV for too long or someone accidently grabs the wrong spoon at the dinner table.

It's easy in late-stage Alzheimer's to become bored with that slow tempo of life, but when I remained open to what was in front of me and not distracted by my thoughts or technology, I usually found Mom waiting there. A memorable experience drove that point home after a doctor's appointment when Mom and I stopped for lunch. I ordered from the menu then took our sandwiches outside and we sat across from each other at a small table.

I was munching away at my sandwich, mindlessly scrolling through my phone. I happened to look up and was almost surprised to see Mom because I was so distracted. But there she was, not eating, just sitting completely still, holding her sandwich and smiling at me—no words—just a warm sweet smile. The moment caught me unaware because I'd almost forgotten she was there, and someday, perhaps sooner than I realized, she would not be. I don't know what she was thinking nor could she have adequately expressed it, but I knew she was present. And I, in my casual indifference to a beautiful moment on a gorgeous day, had my head in the cloud, so to speak, scrolling through social media. I made a vow that day to honor the life that was very much in front of me by being fully present whenever I was with her.

Living in the moment with Mom allowed me to see her in so many ways. She was there in the tender way she helped Lucy out of her chair, in her lightheartedness as she skipped down the hall, and in her voice as she belted out "God Bless America" or other hardwired songs. I saw *her* in her eyes as they twinkled when I entered a room, not remembering I was her daughter but still so happy to see me—whoever I was to her that day. I saw her selfless spirit when she'd offer another resident her dessert if they didn't receive one. Mom loved her dessert.

At night, helping her as she lowered her cumbersome body to kneel in prayer, placing her hands together as she turned her chin and eyes upward, I saw not only the well-worn habits of a religious ritual but also the faith of a daughter calling out to her Father, who heard the prayers she could no longer communicate. As I quietly watched her body remember a revered stance I'd witnessed since childhood, those moments became steeped in an unexplainable holiness—a hallowed place. I sensed a deeper clarity of an uninterrupted connection despite a failed brain.

Although many of these individuals were in the closing moments of their dark night, there was wisdom in the stillness of their days. At times it was so quiet sitting with the residents in the common area that I could almost hear a pin drop. It was in those moments I was tempted to grab my phone or a book to escape what appeared to be emptiness—to fill that void with something—if nothing else, just to pass the time because it moved so slowly. But in fighting off the urge to distract myself, I uncovered a strange type of comfort in that space; in the simple act of holding Mom's hand or watching residents calmly cutting pages from a magazine and gluing then into a collage. There was, astonishingly, a sense that everything was exactly as it should be.

Mom was now moving slower, and she began to nap during the day. For the first time in her life, she was content to just sit. I'd waited my whole life for that and occasionally took it as an opportunity to tell her everything that was happening in my life as well as my boys' and brothers' lives. She didn't jump up to clean dishes or do laundry. She was still, and I imagined her really hearing me as she watched me babble on. She just smiled, and I finally had my mom's full and undivided attention regardless of whether she understood what I was saying. She was in a good space, a reminder of the wise words spoken in my first support group.

The world was quiet there.

Chapter Twenty-Eight

A Word about Fear

Fear cuts deeper than swords.
George R.R. Martin

Like many traits within families, fear can be generational, and I was certain it was in my DNA. Mom's fear crippled her ability to plan for a potential future with Alzheimer's, and I was hostage to similar phobias. Walking away from my grandmother's crying out as I left her imprinted a wound on my psyche not easily erased. Mom and I weren't alone in that fear. According to the Milken Institute, "Adults in the US fear Alzheimer's disease more than cancer, stroke, and heart disease combined."[43]

We live in a results-based and ultra-cognitive society. Combine the loss of cognitive function with the inability to care for oneself and it creates a subculture of individuals much of society deems worthless. Because of declining mental capacities, they land at the mercy of family or friends and their definition of what constitutes a valuable life, including when that life ends. That's a very vulnerable and potentially terrifying position to be in, depending on who makes those decisions. The question of individual worthiness isn't a new one, as history has made clear, and our understanding of humanity painfully evolves.

When I first toured the memory care unit, I was aware of danger not from a safety perspective but from the powerless position in which the individuals there existed. I knew I couldn't stop Mom's runaway train from plowing into it; that was an inevitable reality short of a medical miracle. But I'd avoided it while she was still dancing her way through assisted living. Instead of confronting that truth, I'd side-stepped it, passing it off to a being much more powerful than I. Praying to, pleading with, and cajoling God, I beseeched Him to let Mom pass peacefully in her sleep so that she wouldn't have to experience a locked unit and I wouldn't have to put her there. It was in everyone's best interest, I communicated sincerely, but especially Mom's.

When it was first suggested that the time had come to move Mom into memory care, perhaps their reasoning in having me tour the unit was that I wouldn't view it much differently. There was a similarity in design of the memory care to the three floors of assisted living, but I would have been blind to assume a similar appearance meant a similar reality to me, or Mom. Claustrophobic as I am, all I saw was no escape, and, from a visitor's perspective, most of the individuals appeared totally out of it. Adding to that anxiety was the sweet lady in the rocker swaying back and forth with her baby doll, gently caressing its head. I could only imagine Mom's reaction to that, and although I am touched when I remember that tender scene today, I was in no way prepared for it then.

During that visit, my chest ached as I glanced around at the sweet souls living out their existence locked in. The chilling script I'd carried for eons was playing out live though not exactly in full color—more like shades of gray—before me. I certainly didn't want to leave Mom there, but, peeling back the layers of my anxiety, I uncovered something deeper that had been gnawing at me since Mom was diagnosed although I didn't want to address it; my personal fear of getting Alzheimer's.

Mom buried her fears behind busyness her entire life. I don't believe she consciously pursued an Alzheimer's prevention plan, if there even was one then, but she inherently followed a lot of today's recommendations to avoid getting or to at least delay the disease. I could debate the many possible reasons for Alzheimer's in my family and try to avoid all of the known risk factors, but that still wouldn't take away the fear I carried. I knew I had to break the familial cycle of avoidance and denial by embracing that fear and the painful memories that caused it.

Refusing to confront it made it worse. It morphed from a fear to a phobia, from a physical reaction to a continually negative state of mind. It weakened my ability to accept Mom's future and possibly my own. I fastened myself to those fears, and they needed to be untied for me to walk free. Mom wasn't ready for memory care when first asked to move, but I knew the day would come, and I had to get her and myself ready. In hindsight, the meeting to discuss Mom moving upstairs kick-started the process.

Getting ready was accepting the truth that Mom's disease was progressing, and she was eventually going to a locked unit. Imagining Mom there—how that looked and felt—before it happened helped to mentally and emotionally prepare for that reality. A lot of people use this exercise for many different situations, and while it's a helpful preparation, it took immersing myself in the memory care environment for a while before my fear of a locked unit faded. When it did, I realized the door was not the barrier that had been holding Mom in—the barrier was my own mind.

I once heard it said that if we want to be happy, let go of what makes us sad. My memories of Ma made me sad and fearful. I can still recall those memories, and her journey will always be remembered as a tragic one, but what's changed is those memories no longer cause me anxiety. The fear factor is gone.

Fear hates when we stand up to it and look it in the eye because it loses its power over us. Life was very different on the inside of the locked door, but it was no longer frightening. I had learned something from Mom that she probably never intended to teach me as I watched her soul rise from the ashes of Alzheimer's to reinvent itself: her life force kept on fighting, even as her memory conceded. That wasn't just true for Mom, but for all those individuals I came across in memory care, who at one time only brought to mind a horrible memory of Ma.

In the absence of that fear, life's moments with Mom, good or bad, unfolded as they should. There was no reason to try to control anything because, when fear left the equation, the motivation to make anything different than it already was left too. That also happened with Mom although by different means. Alzheimer's cleared her mind of all the anxiety that came from remembering the past, and that left her more peaceful!

Fear is like waiting in a dentist's chair for a root canal, which studies have proven creates as much mental pain as the physical pain of the procedure itself. I came across a writing once; it was a metaphor to the effect of, "You heal a wound by the blood of that wound." I smeared myself with the blood of my fear. It didn't change any course of action with Mom, and it might not change any future possibilities for me, but it did change my outlook as I realized that fear only serves one purpose, and that is to get us out of danger. Anything short of that only inhibits.

How could I stay out of danger with Alzheimer's? A cure would be a good start, but, for now, keeping up with the latest literature and research and making sure my lifestyle enriches the overall health of my mind, spirit, and body will not only give me the best chance of living a long life, but also a healthy life. The worst-case scenario is that I forget this life I am currently living. Having faith that whoever assumes the role of caregiver will believe I still exist within the stranger that I have become gives me a sword to fight back the fear!

Chapter Twenty-Nine

From the Physical to the Spiritual

Late 2013

We all have that divine moment, when our lives are transformed by the knowledge of the truth.
Lailah Gifty Akita

Mom was in agony. I was out of town when a member of the staff called to let me know that in the past week Lucy had declined rapidly and was dying. They informed me that in the last several days, as Lucy was surrounded by family and hospice, Mom was relentlessly knocking at her door, trying to gain access. The staff were doing their best to distract her, but she had to pass Lucy's room to and from the common areas many times a day.

Mom was banging on doors again, but this time trying to be with Lucy. She was determined, so, short of locking her in her room, they couldn't keep a continual eye on her. Every time the staff thought she was settled in the common area, she was back at Lucy's door. I told them I was five hundred miles away by car but could be back in a day. I couldn't get that heartbreaking image of Mom banging at Lucy's door out of my mind. I felt for Lucy's family, losing that precious soul, and I know they understood Mom's plight, but I have sat with individuals as they lay dying, and I know the necessity for peace in those final, fragile moments. Mom couldn't absorb the concept of death—all she wanted was to be with Lucy. Her confusion and abandonment must have been overwhelming as she was redirected, again and again.

Lucy died within a day of my receiving that call. Mom shed no tears as she was never told; she wouldn't have understood that concept. Her beloved Lucy was just gone. She couldn't have communicated her feelings either; her verbal skills over the past months had deteriorated significantly. She did, however, display the inaudible signs of grief in the following months that Henry Wadsworth Longfellow described perfectly: "There is no grief like the grief that does not speak."

Her appetite declined to the point where she lost a significant amount of weight, and, for the first time in her life, Mom spent a good part of the day on the community couch, sleeping. We gave her appetite stimulants to bulk up her weight, which helped some, but she seemed to have lost her love for food, even ice cream. She wasn't drinking enough fluids and eventually became dehydrated, ending up in the hospital with a bladder infection. Mom wasn't angry or acting out after Lucy's death, but she displayed a flat affect and her eyes were lifeless.

Because of continued weight loss, lack of appetite, despondent state, and Mom's overall decline, the head nurse suggested we enlist the services of hospice. In the spring following Lucy's death, a team arrived with a full array of supportive services for Mom and counseling for me. This is truly a gift of unimaginable proportions not only from a financial perspective as hospice stepped in at this point and covered everything from supplies to palliative medications, but also brought a team of nurses, doctors, social workers, chaplains, music therapy, and volunteers. From my experiences with Mom and other loved ones, this type of caregiving seems to be the true calling of individuals in every area of the hospice team. Although hearing that someone is under the care of hospice does signal the onset of the end, that length of time varies from person to person and is reevaluated every six months.

I assumed Mom, like many others upon signing on with hospice, was months away from passing. But once again, she fought her way back. Although she never completely regained her exuberance, a peaceful disposition reigned, and she began participating once again in activities. The sparkle in her eyes slowly replaced the void left after Lucy's passing. The summer was quiet and peaceful, and we spent many afternoons on the enclosed porch reciting the rosary as she dozed off. As she catnapped between Our Fathers and Hail Marys, I knew those prayers continued on the other side of her peaceful slumber.

In the fall of that year, I noticed Mom disengaging from me. It was slight but palpable. Our relationship had undergone many changes during this journey, but we were now on the edge of another. She wasn't ignoring me or refusing to communicate, but I sensed her movement inward as if to sever the ties that bound her to this earthly existence. I recalled a similar feeling as each of my kids prepared to leave home for college—a sensation of unraveling the symbolic umbilical cord that held us physically close. Yet another aspect of letting go, this one opened to an entirely different way of experiencing Mom. When I looked at her, I still saw a mother's face, but, paralleling her shift, a change was occurring within me as I teetered on the threshold of physically seeing her to spiritually feeling her.

Often, arriving early in the morning before Mom awoke and the staff began their morning rounds, I'd sit silently at the side of her bed. Careful not to disturb her slumber, I'd watch her chest rise and fall in steady rhythms. I wondered if she was dreaming in that peaceful state and if in that altered state of consciousness she was whole in her mind and body. I prayed she was. I found Mom in those few undisturbed moments of tranquility as I became conscious of an unfamiliar awareness. In that somewhere space between our souls, my presence must have collided with hers. As if on cue, Mom would roll her head toward me, slowly open those beautiful blue eyes, and smile as her eyes locked on to mine. There, in that reduced state of electrical activity before her brain stirred and the realities of Alzheimer's surfaced, her eyes exuded presence, and her sweet smile communicated everything that her cognitive state could not.

I held her gaze and returned that smile, knowing with every ounce of my being that we were connecting on a level that transcended our human existence and comprehension, inhabiting that space without form where our physical bodies lose their separate entities and our souls converge like separate rivers arriving at a juncture then flowing together. Those undisturbed moments of quietude were void of the usual clamoring and busyness of my mind, creating the opening for an unspoken but extraordinary communication—and I knew in that instant that I was known by my mom.

Chapter Thirty

If It Gets Too Tough, Mom, It's OK to Let Go

Thanksgiving 2014

*The old man smiled. "I shall not die of a cold, my son.
I shall die of having lived."*
Willa Cather

Shortly before Thanksgiving of that same year, I received another summons to appear before the administrative staff. Memory care held quarterly care planning meetings between a member of the nursing staff and the family of the resident. At these meetings, medications, psychosocial wellbeing, nutritional status, and behavior issues were discussed. Any questions or concerns were also addressed.

Mom had been under hospice care for the better part of that year. I was certain they wanted to talk about her decline, so I prepared myself for any actions they wanted to take. Assuming I might be asked to further augment her care, I pre-emptively investigated hiring an aide to stay with Mom during the times when neither hospice nor I was there.

During the weekdays, the activities director, Laurel, kept the residents busy and stimulated for most of the day. Mom was very content in that space and went along with whatever was planned, as she had developed a very special connection with Laurel. After breakfast, I would push Mom's wheelchair over to the large table where Laurel was setting up crafts and other activities for the residents. Confident that she was in good hands, I was free to run errands, or go for a swim. I was in and out during the day, so there were gaps—mostly during the evenings and especially at dinner—where there were not enough aides to help with all the residents who needed assistance.

At the time I was asked to attend the meeting, I was aware of the depth of Mom's decline. She had developed a stubborn stage two pressure sore on her lower leg, which was under control but not abating. In the months leading up to this meeting she'd made a big backward transition, moving from a walker to a wheelchair. Mealtimes had become increasingly difficult as she was disinterested in a lot of the foods she normally enjoyed. She sometimes needed cues to eat by herself and other times needed to be fed.

Individuals with Alzheimer's lose their sense of smell, and one of the effects of that is loss of appetite. Mom was mostly interested in soft foods like scrambled eggs, oatmeal, mashed potatoes, pudding, and, of course, ice cream. Her verbal skills were by now limited to a few words, mostly yes and no but also STOP, in the loudest voice she could muster when a caregiver or I assisted her with something she didn't want to do. Her bladder incontinence also worsened, and she required full assistance with bathing and dressing.

Hours before the morning meeting, I noticed Mom was moving her mouth as if she was chewing gum. This was something new, and I was concerned that she had a loose tooth or something foreign in her mouth. When I asked her to open her mouth, I noticed she had leftover food from breakfast in her cheeks. I immediately reported this to the nurse in charge who checked Mom and informed me she was "pocketing" food.

I wasn't familiar with the term, but what I came to learn is that this odd occurrence is a late-stage symptom where the individual holds food in their cheeks or under their tongue. They do this because they are forgetting how and when to swallow. As more food goes into their mouth and they don't swallow, the food gets stored, which then creates a choking hazard. Mom still had the ability to swallow because she was still eating and digesting food but was sometimes forgetting, and that's when food would be pocketed. There are different ways to assist with this situation, such as verbal prompts to swallow between mouthfuls. The easiest solution though was to pulverize the food and thicken the liquids so that Mom didn't choke.

Despite all her worsening issues, Mom never spent a day in bed. She was up and dressed every day and seemed satisfied whether she participated in the group activities, or just watched the others. I didn't know her timeline, but I learned from her hospice nurse that this phase of physical decline could speed up—or perhaps pause for quite a while. Timetables are unique to everyone. But there was something deep in my being—a feeling I couldn't adequately verbalize but knew for certain—Mom was, in the words of Cincinnati MLB legend, Joe Nuxhall,[44] "Rounding third and heading for home." Mom and I were sharing a fragile space, suspended in that delicate domain between a fading fall leaf separating from the branch and its slow and graceful dance toward earth. It was the space where we hold on tight to what we have always known because we know we must let it go. I could physically feel the impending split.

Mom's last care plan meeting had been in late October. There, we discussed the pressure sore, which was being treated by her hospice nurse three times a week. Other than that, I signed off on her current meds and for her care plan to continue. This unscheduled request came mid-November, just a week before Thanksgiving.

I remember the morning well because I was planning for our annual Biggs/Benz Thanksgiving celebration when the call came in. Most of my siblings and their families drove in from Cincinnati and Florida. These were crazy, fun, and loud gatherings when Mom, her kids, and their families settled into our home for the long holiday weekend. Moving Mom to Georgia full time became even more reason for the extended family to road trip it to Atlanta.

Deep into that planning, I was distracted by that sense of separation I was feeling with Mom. I'd first noticed Mom distancing herself almost exactly a year earlier when the family was in for Thanksgiving. Sometime during that holiday, we had a tradition of decorating Mom's room for Christmas. She lived for holidays and birthdays—really any reason to celebrate. These observances were steeped in rich traditions but none more so than Christmas.

Growing up, Mom made Christmas magical. There were pine wreaths with big red bows adorning the doors, electric candles in the windows, ceramic lighted Christmas trees on tabletops, big multicolored light bulbs framing the house, and, of course, the ever-growing collection of Dickens' Christmas Villages. Christmas cookies were placed in tins and hidden in the cloak closet in the hope they'd make it to Christmas Eve. In our living room the tall artificial Christmas tree held center stage in front of a large picture window, brimming with multicolored glass balls, assorted ornaments, lights, and tons of tinsel. A rustic wooden shelter sat under the tree with stable animals hovering close to the makeshift inn. Inside, Mary and Joseph positioned themselves around a tiny feeding box filled with hay. They kneeled as they waited for baby Jesus to arrive. A beautiful angel hung at the apex of that stable, watching over this young Jewish family.

If you journeyed alongside of us during the Christmas season, the first stop was The Baker House in Oxford, Ohio, where we sipped hot cocoa and purchased hand-crafted wooden ornaments.

There was a day of cookie making, many days of shopping, and a night at the Aronoff Center, watching the *Nutcracker* ballet. The grand finale was Christmas Eve dinner and a visit from old Santa himself, who doled out early gifts for the kids and grandkids. For those still awake, Midnight Mass with an hour of Christmas carols prior awaited. Mom loved every minute of it and joyfully anticipated and began planning for this festive season soon after the Thanksgiving feast ended.

The Christmas season with all its trappings and traditions continued to captivate Mom up until moderate dementia, but we had to adjust our plans to accommodate her ever-changing condition. While she once loved the hustle and bustle of the season's activities, she became more agitated and confused when she experienced large crowds, bright lights, and loud noises. She stressed when she was away from the retirement community for long periods, often pleading to go home.

After moving Mom into memory care, we stopped taking her out for these holiday events, but decorating her room was still a real treat for her, even if she couldn't remember the reason for the frivolity or everyone's name. She reveled in the merrymaking and actively participated in the tree trimming.

That was true up until a year ago when I sensed a remoteness in her while decorating her room for Christmas. She became an observer as she watched from the sidelines, indifferent to the fun and slipping out of the room to join other residents in the common area. I would bring her back, but before long she would leave again. Clearly her comfort zone resided in the familiarity of her memory care family. While there was consolation in that, there was an ongoing tug at my heart as another layer of our shared bond was being stripped away.

By this time, I thought I was immune to the changes that Alzheimer's continually threw at me, believing that I could somehow avoid the emotional roller coaster through knowledge of what was coming. But over the course of Mom's last year, and especially since Lucy's death, I'd been continually sad, and my tears flowed at the most random and inopportune times. I attributed it to being tired. Expressing this feeling to the hospice chaplain, I was told this state of mind is called "anticipatory grief."[45] I was grieving Mom's passing from this earth before it happened, and this occurs with many diseases, such as dementias and incurable cancers.

This gloom surrounded me like a dark cloud on the morning of my meeting. I don't envy the bearer of bad news, and it's a position no one wants to be in, but unfortunately it coincides with certain occupations. Most of us at some moments have been on the receiving side of that desk, door, or phone call when unpleasant news is delivered. I'd been there before and was ready for a challenging conversation, but, once again, I was not prepared for the bomb that was dropped on me.

Assisted living and memory care had become our family for the past three and a half years. The physical building housed Mom, but inside the brick and mortar, her life and mine, to a large extent during that time, were interwoven with other residents, family members, and staff. This was her sanctuary. Her daily routines provided stability, and the familiar faces she encountered calmed her mind and gave her peace in a world full of uncertainty and confusion. This place—so far in terms of distance and every other way from the home she'd left in Cincinnati when she'd first moved in with me—now embodied home for her, and I had come to rely on the support of the family members and staff of this community as we laughed and cried while traversing the rugged terrain of Alzheimer's.

Within those walls I'd witnessed the extremes of compassion, love, and abandonment, but mostly profound tenderness between staff, family members, and their loved ones. Dementia was the thread that braided together individuals who would have never otherwise crossed paths. Our commonality created a safe harbor in which to dwell. Despite Mom's now rapidly deteriorating inner condition, she was sheltered, loved, and protected. I had peace in the assumption that when she was finally called home, she would not only be surrounded by her biological family but also by this current family.

"We are so sorry, your mom has been here a long time, but due to her immobility we must ask her to leave . . . couldn't get her out in a fire . . . concerned about her choking . . . a liability . . . so sorry. This is so hard; we all love your mom . . . she needs to be out in a month. We will make some calls for you, let us know if there is anything we can do."

There may have been more said, but my mind was focused on "out"—they were throwing her out. My sweet, vulnerable, and fragile mom was being asked to leave her haven, and at a critical juncture in her journey. My grandmother's illness had been mishandled near the beginning, and now Mom's was being mishandled near the end.

A dream replayed in my mind. A baby was crawling in the dark, alongside the road as I drove by. I slammed my foot on the brake, but the car would not stop. I tried to open the door and jump from the car, but the door was stuck. I screamed as I looked back, seeing that tiny baby become smaller and smaller as the car continued to advance farther away.

This was a reoccurring dream I experienced after my first son was born. I would wake in terror, leap out of bed, and sprint to the nursery as fast as my feet would allow. Bursting into his room further roused me from that semi-conscious state, but there I always found him—safe and sound.

Sitting motionless in that office chair, I realized Mom was now that baby. She was exposed to the dark night and susceptible to the dangers lurking around her, and I couldn't stop the car. She kept getting smaller and smaller. The stormy dark clouds that had surrounded me for months opened, and a deluge of torrential rains pelted down, on my face, and over the edge of the dam. Below it, Mom's sanctuary was being washed away.

I left the meeting, reeling from the blow. I can't ever recall feeling so powerless, afraid, and rejected. I found Mom sitting in her wheelchair alongside the other residents at the craft table in the living room. Laurel was having them cut out pictures in magazines. Soft music was playing in the background. I remember thinking it was someone from the Rat Pack, a familiar sound for many of the residents although no longer a household name for most. Regardless, a voice that brought comfort through its familiarity. It was just another normal day in memory care. Except for us.

I avoided making eye contact with anyone as I approached Mom. Quietly, I wheeled her away from the table and led her down the hall and into her room. I took in her handsome studio apartment. Outside of the house in Cincinnati, this was the only other place Mom had considered home in the last fifty-five years.

My eyes fell on the beautiful dark-gold patterned window treatments and bedding my sister-in-law so lovingly created. I observed the sitting area with her comfortable overstuffed chairs, and the hutch that housed some of her lifelong and beloved figurines and treasures. Mom's wedding album, which up until the past year she'd proudly shared with everyone who came into her room, sat on the coffee table. She could no longer identify the individuals in the album, but she continued to look through it, slowly turning the pages and gazing at the nearly seventy-year-old photographs.

I thought about the many times when I couldn't find the album in her room, especially when she was in assisted living. I'd search all the areas Mom frequented and eventually locate it on a coffee table in the main lobby or in Lucy's room. She often carried it with her then left it behind when she got distracted. She had an emotional attachment to that album, well beyond the point where she could tell you why.

I glanced at the walls, covered with pictures of her family, past and present. When Mom first moved into assisted living she would point to and identify each person in the photographs, and there were a lot of people to keep track of with six kids, eighteen grandkids, and a few great grandkids. This room was what remained of her earthly life, her eighty-nine-year-old legacy consolidated into a fifteen-by-fifteen space. It was nearly identical to the room she'd occupied one floor below when in assisted living.

I pulled her wheelchair over to a chair, sitting down to face her. As I often did, I asked her who I was. She answered in a soft and barely audible voice, "Marianne." I told her that I loved her. She nodded, then slowly repeated the word "love" back to me in a soft whisper. Her voice, especially in the past few months, had gradually lost its force and was now faint and weak. Her vocabulary was limited to a few words, usually singular. I looked into her eyes—they were tired but still that brilliant aquamarine blue.

I quietly told her that we were going to take a trip. Mom had been an avid traveler, and I often used this strategy when we had to leave the building for a doctor's appointment, especially over the past half year as she grew increasingly afraid to leave her familiar surroundings. A trip—the irony of that statement caught me unexpectedly as I realized that a trip was something you usually returned from. In that moment, the full implication of the meeting's ugly truth came thundering down all around me. *Where would we go? Who would take Mom in her present state?*

Could she survive a move? Why, like so many other residents in memory care, wasn't she able to live out her life here? How could we start over? And why? Why this? Why now?

My heart broke for her, and the precarious situation we were in. In hindsight, I should have moved her to an establishment that legally guaranteed her the ability to age—and die—in place. Instead, I took for granted what I'd been told three and a half years earlier, that, unless she required specialized nursing care that hospice couldn't supply, she would never have to leave. I was told that most patients ended up in hospice and died there. Indeed, most, if not all, of the residents I had known during Mom's tenure in memory care had followed that path.

I had no idea when Mom's time would be up or if she was close. I knew she was exhibiting many of the final symptoms of late-stage Alzheimer's, but even a patient with all the final symptoms can linger in late stage for quite a while. What I did know was what this move would do to her.

I stared at Mom, so childlike and vulnerable, and in that instant, I decided. I wanted her to know that when it got too tough and if she was ready, she could stop fighting. I intuitively knew that even if she could not understand my words, her heart could discern my message.

I inhaled slowly and looked deeply into her beautiful eyes. I felt that non-verbal communication of unconditional love between us. We had always been honest and looked out for each other's best interests. We had our differences and at times we drove each other crazy, but our bond was absolute and unbreakable.

I took Mom's beautiful, weathered old hands into mine—good strong hands that had raised six kids. Hands that cooked and cleaned and dressed and fed. Hands that held and hugged and applauded. Hands that colored and painted and built sandcastles with grandchildren and great grandchildren. I clasped those ancient hands that had tenderly cared for my dad during his battle with colon cancer and championed Ma through her journey with Alzheimer's. Those lovely, sturdy, and capable hands that saw babies in and loved ones out.

"I've loved you, Mom, every day of my life for as long as I can remember." Wiping my wet cheeks with my sleeve, I continued. "You were such a good and faithful wife to Dad and did such a great job of raising all six of us kids." Mom was so still—her eyes locked on to mine as she watched me intently. I went on. "I am so proud of how you cared for Dad when he was sick and courageously fought for Ma, and I know how hard you battled this beast when you started to forget things." I tightened my grip on her hands. "I want you to know that I've tried my very best to take care of you, and every decision I've made, as hard as it may have been for you at times, was always with your best interests at heart." I looked down before I continued, digging deep for the courage to express the words that I knew were going to break my heart even further and maybe hers too. "You've fought the good fight, Mom, throughout this disease, and I know how hard you tried to get me to see you. I see you Mom—I always did." I took another deep breath and continued. "Things might get tough again, and I want you to know that no one will blame you if you've had enough and are ready to give up. I will miss you every day, but I'll be OK."

Mom's hands began to shake as she tried to gesture something in her late-stage, non-verbal form of communication. I released her hands from mine. Slowly, she raised her arms, quivering as they were, up to my face. Her trembling, familiar old hand cradled my cheek as the other tried to wipe away my tears. There, in that that moment, we were transported back in time. I was that child who had scraped my knee, the teenager whose heart was broken for the first time, and the young mother who had just lost her dad to cancer.

Her desire to comfort was still present within the thick and cumbersome walls of dementia, and that deep indwelling source of love broke through and sprang forth to offer solace. Whether or not Mom understood our relationship to each other, her actions on that traumatizing day spoke volumes for the words that failed her. She became a mom again, comforting a daughter. She was a fighter and still had something to say. Her spirit remained resplendent, even in her brokenness, softly echoing messages of love from the depths of her soul.

I don't know if Mom was quite ready to let go or not, but I did know that it was her decision. She never liked being told what to do, but as we were embarking on a new journey that promised to be difficult in her weakened condition, I wanted her to know that if the going got too tough, it was OK for her to let go.

Chapter Thirty-One

No Room at the Inn

November 2014

All God's angels come to us disguised.
James Russell Lowell

I wheeled Mom to the common area where the activities director was working with other residents, and pushed her in close to the table. Glancing up, I caught Laurel's attention. Her brows arched into a questioning expression; it was obvious by my red, swollen eyes that something was amiss. I glanced away. My mind was spiraling out of control, and I had to get out of there and quick. I gave mom a hug and bolted. I was on the clock.

T-minus thirty days to find a place that would take Mom in her condition and move her in. It felt like I had to move a mountain, and that, as I would come to find out, may have been easier. I left the building and scrambled for my keys as I headed toward my truck. Climbing in, I stared down at my phone then up to Mom's room. As I continued to stare, a video launched in my mind that recalled happier times as well as the fun whenever my husband and brothers were together, teasing mom, dancing with her, and acting silly. They could always get her laughing.

I remembered the wonder in her eyes, like those of a child, wide with excitement as she took in the twinkling lights on the tree and the frosty white snowman cycling seasonal colors. We set all the lights to go off at dusk and on at dawn so that she could close her eyes in that tranquil scene and open them back up to the magic. I thought about the tree trimming party from the previous year, recalling the separation and loneliness I sensed in her, even amidst the tight, loving family that surrounded her. Now I wondered where she would be celebrating Christmas this year.

I was sidetracked in my daydream by a car that pulled in abruptly next to mine. Disentangling myself from those memories as I wiped my eyes, I looked back to my phone. Frantically I googled memory units and nursing facilities within a twenty-five-mile radius of my home. A few miles in parts of Atlanta could take half an hour to drive at certain times of day, even an hour in areas of town that are closer to the city center. I wanted to be close enough so that I could get to her fast and not spend half of my day driving.

Soon I had a list and started my calls. I also phoned some friends whose parents were in memory care or nursing units nearby to see if they had any pull in getting Mom in quick. Most reputable facilities have waiting lists, so the vast number of my options were eliminated immediately. Many others did not want to take Mom for the same reason she was being discharged. I would have taken her home with me, but three years after she'd moved out, we'd renovated our first-floor bathroom, removing all the handicapped-accessible bars in the process. My home was now not suitable for someone in Mom's condition for a multitude of reasons, the biggest being the layout of our main level bathroom. It couldn't accommodate a wheelchair, plus there wasn't enough room between the toilet and shower for Mom and the person she'd need to assist her. I was therefore at the mercy of an establishment to accept Mom. I knew the odds of finding a place within a reasonable drive from my home were slim, and I started to panic as the full implication hit me head on—I really had no place to take her.

There was only one nursing home within my search that could accommodate Mom immediately—twenty-two miles from my home. But I had to consider it as there were no other openings and no time to waste. They were able to see me that evening. As I drove onto the property, I thought the outside of the building and the grounds were pretty although that wouldn't matter to Mom at this point. I parked in front of the nursing home and entered the small lobby. The receptionist was sweet and compassionate as I told her Mom's story. Someone came out to give me a tour, and my heart quickly sank as I walked through the building, passing residents lined up on either side of the halls in their wheelchairs. Some were asleep sitting up and some slouched over. It brought back painful memories of my grandmother and once again I fought back tears. I knew I couldn't leave Mom there. Still, after the tour, I followed my guide to the sales office and began to initiate paperwork but stopped—I just couldn't do it. I abruptly left the facility, shaken but determined, and continued to make calls.

Over the next couple of days, I arranged appointments with staff nurses at four prospective memory care facilities to come and interview Mom. I had no idea what type of heartache that would become as I watched, one by one, all four regretfully decline to take Mom "in her condition." Mom was beginning to pocket food, but that was not the big deterrent because most of these places would pulverize her meals.

The main issue was she was not able to ambulate forward in her wheelchair. She could move her chair backward by pushing off with her feet, but she wasn't able to move her feet in a forward walking motion to propel the chair forward. She had either forgotten how to do it or lost the muscle strength it required, or perhaps both. I understood the importance of moving oneself forward in the event of a fire, especially if there weren't enough staff present to assist residents who couldn't get themselves out. I doubted very seriously that any place, even a nursing home, had a 1:1 ratio of staff to non-ambulatory residents, even though that was their stipulation.

Now I had to get creative. I called the establishments back that had declined Mom, asking if they would reconsider with a range of options I suggested. I presented several scenarios—from round-the-clock aides to practically moving in with her. They still wouldn't budge. When I called Sun-Up Assisted Living, which was located across from my neighborhood, I spoke with the head nurse, Juli. As I begged her to please give Mom a second chance, the phone went silent. I was about to ask if she was still there when she spoke up and agreed to come out herself and give Mom another look. We set up a time for her to meet us. I was cautiously optimistic.

On the morning of the meeting, my husband and I went over early to help the hospice nurse bathe and dress Mom. We picked out a soft pink top and I curled her hair. I brushed some color on her cheeks and applied her favorite pink lipstick. We then set out to practice moving forward in her chair. As we had done every day since Juli agreed to come visit, we placed Mom's feet on the floor and simulated a walking motion. We then asked her to repeat the motion and move toward us. She was close but couldn't quite do it herself. She was great at moving backward and could back out of the room with no problem, but she was sadly unable to move her chair forward.

When did this happen? I usually pushed her in the wheelchair but not because I thought she couldn't do it herself, more as a convenience. I racked my brain trying to remember the last time she was able to move forward independently. There just wasn't an obvious end point. But even if there had been, would it have made any difference? I still wouldn't have known that the criteria for her to remain in memory care was to ambulate forward in her wheelchair. Tears welled up.

Juli arrived late morning and began her assessment. Steve and I stood by anxiously as she talked to Mom, took her vitals, and examined the sore on her leg. Mom was responding well to Juli; her eyes were clear and bright, and she was smiling. Juli then asked Mom if she could move her chair toward her. The moment of truth had arrived. We'd done everything humanly possible, so now I prayed, "God, let her move that chair forward, just give her Your strength to do whatever it takes."

Steve and I stood behind Juli, as she sat facing Mom, and enthusiastically prompted Mom to move toward us, just as we'd encouraged our three boys to take their first steps decades earlier. Mom had her own cheerleading team, and she was looking up at us, smiling, happy to be the center of such positive attention. Juli asked her to try again, and then again. The tone in our voices began to change as we went from cheering to pleading. Emotion engulfed us, even Juli, and I could hear in her voice the desire for Mom to move. We were becoming desperate.

Juli was patient and gave Mom many opportunities, but she simply couldn't move forward. My heart was sinking as I felt the door closing. Then Juli leaned forward and looked into Mom's eyes as she placed her hand on Mom's knee. She very tenderly asked her to move forward. Steve walked around and butted up against the back of Mom's chair. I held my breath for what seemed like an eternity. Mom's chair moved, ever so slightly, but it moved. I looked at Steve. We looked at Juli. Did she see it? Was it enough? Time stood still.

Juli then looked up at us and uttered words that elevated the terms mercy and compassion to a new altitude, "We can care for your mom."

Steve and I immediately hugged each other, and then we hugged Juli. We were overjoyed. It seemed as if we'd just won the lottery. We made plans to move Mom the Monday following the upcoming Thanksgiving weekend.

Juli's response to our desperate dilemma will be forever implanted in my heart. By agreeing to take Mom in her condition, she breathed life into a vulnerable and broken old woman who had been told there was no room at the inn. Mom had a new home, and sitting at the apex of that stable was as angel disguised as a human. Her name was Juli.

Chapter Thirty-Two

The Gang's All Here

Thanksgiving Week 2014

*The strength of a family, like the strength of an army,
lies in its loyalty to each other.*
Mario Puzo

Kevin and Cathy were the first to arrive for the Thanksgiving celebration. It was the Wednesday before Thanksgiving, and they were meeting Steve and me in Mom's room. Mom had a late afternoon hair appointment, and the four of us escorted her to the second floor where the salon was located. The stylist there had been doing Mom's hair for most of her tenure in memory care, but since Mom had become wheelchair bound the process was much more complex.

This feat was a labor of love for the stylist as she pulled the heavy salon chair out from under the sink and pushed Mom's wheelchair up to the basin to wash her hair. The chair was not a perfect fit, so she wrapped Mom's neck and shoulders in plastic and used numerous towels around and under her to try to ensure she did not get soaked, which she sometimes still did.

After the wash she'd roll Mom's hair and transport her to the dryer. We would both help Mom into the dryer chair and lower the cap over her head. At this point Mom was usually exhausted and asleep within minutes. When her hair was dry, we would help her back into the wheelchair and set her in front of the mirror where the stylist would finish up combing out Mom's curls and styling her hair.

This process may seem like too much for someone at this point in their disease, but, when Mom's hair was finished and she looked at her reflection in the mirror, what stared back was a pretty lady with soft, beautiful white curls and a big smile on her face. That beam made all the effort worthwhile. This day before Thanksgiving was no different, and Mom was glowing from her new cut and style. Her nails had been painted a few days earlier, and she was ready for the festive holiday celebrations!

The rest of the family arrived during the afternoon and evening, and Mom was surrounded all weekend by her kids and grandkids. It's not easy to continue travelling hours and hours, year after year, with kids and dogs when the major reason for your visit stops remembering you. I think it's even harder for family members who don't experience the day-to-day decline in their loved ones. For me, the pieces that slowly fell away allowed me to grieve bit by bit. When my siblings saw Mom, they were hit with massive changes that were a shock to their system.

But the grandkids took it all in stride. There is nothing quite like witnessing the ease with which they love, even when it's difficult. Mom had declined quite a bit since most of the out-of-town grandkids had last seen her. I knew seeing her this way was hard for them, especially witnessing her weakness and fragility. Mom had never been weak, and, even in her dementia, she'd remained strong-spirited and fun for so long. I watched them surround her that weekend, sharing their stories of school and jobs.

Drew, our youngest, was excited to share his medical school acceptances with her. "Memaw," he proudly exclaimed, "I'm in!" while others showed her pictures and videos on their phones—getting her to smile and laugh! I watched her demeanor change as these grandkids showered her with affection, and it was in those precious moments that I came to fully understand the healing power of reciprocal generational love.

Her advanced dementia and inability to communicate didn't deter this group of teenagers and young adults as they lovingly interacted with her, and she, through her responsiveness in the form of smiles and laughter, reciprocated. Over the years, all the grandkids had reaped the benefits of her guidance and insight and observed her ability to have fun and never let her age define her, but that was nothing compared to the pure gift of unconditional love she rained on them.

Mom in return allowed them to keep her young. She was always one of the last to bed at night when different families gathered under one roof, chatting away the hours. At weddings and family events, she was consistently part of the lingering few still left on the dance floor for the last few songs—the others were her grandkids. They profited from and enjoyed each other immensely!

The gang surrounded Mom on what was to become her final Thanksgiving. There was strength and beauty in this big extended family, and those attributes existed solely because of the loyalty of its members. Mom would have been so proud!

Chapter Thirty-Three

Moving Day, Monday

December 1, 2014

Life is made of so many partings welded together.
Charles Dickens

The Thanksgiving holiday flew by, and most of the family gathered early Sunday morning for one last picture with Mom before going their separate ways. Goodbyes are always emotional for me, but this parting was especially poignant. The weekend was fun and a great distraction, but, just as soon as everyone left, the heaviness I'd been experiencing over both Mom's accelerating decline and her impending move returned and nearly flattened me.

I was anxious about moving Mom the next day, especially because my boys had returned either to college or their home in another state, and Steve was out of town. I was on my own, and while normally that wouldn't bother me, I couldn't shake a lingering sense of dread. I was cloaked in a dark cloud and at times found it hard to breathe.

Monday morning arrived as a clear sunny day, and I was grateful. I knew clouds and rain would have amplified my melancholy. I got to memory care early, before Mom was awake, and sat next to her bed as she slept. She was peaceful in that somewhere realm that exists beyond our conscious state, and, as I watched her, I wished she could remain there forever.

I had no idea what to expect from the day. I knew I didn't want to say goodbye to all the kind souls who had become my family. I especially didn't want Mom in her weakened state to start all over with individuals who did not know her and love her. I wanted Mom to live out her days in the familiarity of her surroundings, encircled by recognizable faces. In her late stage of dementia, any change in the routine, even as minor as switching who she sat next to at the dining table, could throw her off. Doctor's appointments, which required leaving the building, frightened her and required additional assistance. She was comforted by consistency and rattled by change.

The hospice nurse arrived, and we bathed and dressed Mom. I wheeled her down to the dining room and helped her eat some oatmeal. She was quiet and peaceful, but of course she didn't know what was coming. The movers arrived mid-morning, and I left her with the group gathered for morning activities. I began packing her belongings into boxes as the movers disassembled and wrapped her furniture.

Family members who were visiting their loved ones drifted in and out of Mom's room during the morning and early afternoon to say their goodbyes and talk about what had happened. I know it was an eye-opening and chilling revelation for them to hear Mom's story: they now understood that this could also happen to them. I felt for them in their fear because they were also at the mercy of a system that could, without warning, evict their loved one at the worst possible time.

So many thoughts ran through my mind that morning as I placed her once-cherished collectables—that now only held memories for me—into bins. This was Mom's home—her supposed final home—and the physical acts of breaking down her material life, removing pictures, folding clothes, and bubble wrapping valuables, allowed me the space to reflect on the myriad possible whys that Mom was being thrown out.

Our experience with the individuals who worked directly with Mom, including nurses, aides, therapists, activities director, and hospice, was that they were competent, loving, and empathetic. The disconnect was in the administration and the director of nursing, who, in my experience and opinion, were detached from the residents and insensitive to the needs of the families.

I had to remind myself that assisted living and memory care communities are businesses first. They provide need-based products because the consumer can no longer live on their own. But unlike nursing homes, they do not fall under federal regulations and, therefore, residents can be evicted. Oversight is at the state level, and there is considerable elasticity within state regulations depending upon how the community is set up and defined. Assisted living communities with memory care facilities are often advertised as offering "continual care" or "aging in place," loose terminology used in sales pitches to entice residents. Today, hospice often bridges the gap for those residents who need more than what memory care can provide but don't require full-scale nursing. Mom was in that gap along with most of the residents who'd passed during her tenure.

The true embodiments of continual care and aging in place are places that will provide care until death, period. And that can only happen in a community attached to a nursing unit. I remembered well the conversation we had with the sales associate before we moved Mom into assisted living. She did say that most of the residents retained hospice at the end and passed there. I understood there was no guarantee that Mom could remain there until she died as we had nothing in writing. But it seemed like a long way off at the time, and I felt we had a type of gentleman's agreement. That was my error.

Driving around our city today, I see endless, beautiful retirement communities popping up without nursing. I am concerned about where all those residents will go when the terms of their stays, loosely defined as they may be, are up. With Mom, Alzheimer's progressed in leaps and lulls. Even if I'd been made aware that we would have to move her at some point, that juncture was—and remains—ill-defined and hazy. There was certainly no warning, no form of oral or written communication implying she was in a declining state that signified or even hinted at a future move. She'd been in hospice, and I had assumed she was safe.

I've learned over time that it's a good idea to put distance between emotionally charged experiences and my response to them. For me, perspective grows in the space between the hedges. Unlike my feisty and strong-willed mom, I don't do well when I'm caught off guard, usually preferring to duck or run until I can gather my thoughts.

When Mom was asked to leave, I was not only unprepared but also in a vulnerable and depressive state because of Mom's declining condition. Looking back, I should have fought harder for Mom to stay and pulled out any cards in my arsenal that may have challenged the administration. Today, the threat of a negative online review might have been enough for them to consider other options for Mom. This is not about the duration of her life; rather, it speaks to the quality of those days and the suffering that she, and consequently we, endured because of her move.

※ ※ ※

The ambulance arrived for Mom as the movers packed the last of her furniture in their truck. I taped up the remaining boxes intended for my truck and met with the floor nurse to sign off on medications and exit paperwork. The movers were following me to her new assisted living facility. Mom was placed on the stretcher in the common area and strapped in. I kissed her goodbye and told her I would see her shortly but hesitated to give her any more information. Not really knowing what she could comprehend, and fearing she might panic with the truth, I chose to leave it there.

Most of the residents were watching the commotion from the large activity table, and a few came over and wanted to know where Mom was going. I told them that she would be back shortly. Francis, a kind gentleman I got to know well and who lived on the assisted living floor walked over to the stretcher. His wife resided in memory care, and he spent his days alongside her. They shared meals, and he participated in the group activities with the rest of us. They often took walks and listened to music and were always holding hands. She napped on his shoulder. The love between them broke through any barrier that her dementia erected. They sat with us at Mom's dining table, and we got to know each other over many meals. He cried as they rolled Mom out. I didn't tell him she was leaving, but he knew she wasn't coming back.

Glancing toward the TV area, I spotted Patrick, a WWII veteran, well-known by his hat, which was bedecked with military decorations and badges. He wore it every day. He was sitting in just about the same spot as on that day when I first reluctantly toured memory care. He didn't move around very much and mostly just sat in a chair. Catching my eye, he smiled as I was leaving, and I am pretty sure he smiled most days across Mom's entire memory care stay. He would shout out a gruff "Hi" as I walked by then flash the biggest smile he could manage. It wouldn't seem this older gentleman, who spent his days in a chair locked behind a door, would have much to be happy about. But he continued to smile, and boy could that ear-to-ear grin lift my spirits. I believe that infectious cheer effected change in the hearts of many of the family members who crossed his sunny path.

Sitting on the couch was Georgia, who was married to Francis. She was a member of her church choir in her previous life and was always singing. She sang a heart-rending rendition of "How Great Thou Art," which always managed to open wide the windows of my being and send my spirit soaring. Her voice was still impressive and strong, but it was her facial expression that captivated me the most, and that image will never leave me. Soon after breaking out in song, she would close her eyes and slowly lift her head, lips curling upward as she released those beautiful lyrics. Then, inhaling deeply before ascending the musical scale to the song's finale, she thundered out a "how great Thou art." I knew those of us listening had fallen away from her at that point for I could see by her expression that she was now singing to an audience of One.

There was an unspoken communion that existed within memory care. This was a unique group of individuals from all different walks of life who didn't choose this path, but, because of their commonality with dementia, they lived, laughed, ate, and socialized together. They shared a baffling bond, but a connection all the same. There were, of course, the occasional squabbles that would be expected in any type of communal living but mostly a genuine affection among individuals who didn't know each other's names yet instinctively knew how to give and receive love.

Their friendships were not based on who they were, how much money they earned, or what they could do for each other because they no longer understood the significance of those things. They were blinded to worldly attachments, freeing them up for the only thing that truly lasts—love—and most of them gave it away with reckless abandon.

I thought back to the first time I set foot in memory care. There was not much outward change from assisted living as I glanced around at the open floor plan, but change occurred and, for me, it was all internal. Little did I know that this small group of individuals locked away from the outside world would forever change my understanding of our existence on this earth. My heart no longer broke for them, who by all outward appearances appeared lost, for I had found the beauty in their brokenness. That transformation didn't come from a book or an inspirational speaker but from immersing myself in the lives of those sidelined souls who appeared irrelevant and disconnected from life. They taught me everything I thought I already knew about life and death, love and loss.

Glancing towards Laurel, I saw she was busy trying to distract the other residents from the situation with Mom's move. She was the real lifeblood of this group, working daily with each resident at their own level yet managing to keep everyone together and happy as a group. I shot one last look around the room that Mom considered home and to the staff and residents who had become our family. I felt their eyes on me. Turning toward that locked door, I entered the code and walked through the same way I'd walked in—some eighteen months earlier—with tears streaming down my face.

Chapter Thirty-Four

A Brief Visit, Sunday

14 December 2014

He who binds to himself a joy,
Does the winged life destroy.
But he who kisses the joy as it flies,
Lives in Eternity's sunrise.
WILLIAM BLAKE

The movers and I arrived mid-afternoon, and I instructed them in the arrangement of Mom's furniture in her studio, which turned out to be in assisted living. There were no available rooms in memory care, but she would still be spending her days with activities and meals there. The room was roughly the same size as her last residence, and there was a nice view from the large window facing the woods. We laid out the furniture in a similar fashion as before, and I was hopeful that once the pictures were on the walls and the treatments on the windows, this would become her new home. A different hospice would be caring for her but performing the same functions. As we were now fewer than two miles from my home, I imagined I would walk there on nice days.

The furniture was in place, clothing hung in the closet and folded in the drawers, and Mom's bed was made. The floor by the window was still strewn with boxes containing pictures and collectables, but that would have to wait until my husband was back in town. I turned on soft music from the radio alarm clock and proceeded to the memory care unit. The tough part was behind us, and I was anxious see Mom.

I walked into memory care and was directed to the kitchen bar area where the residents in wheelchairs were being served dinner. I asked about Mom, and someone pointed me in the direction of a wheelchair. I walked toward her but suddenly stopped.

One of the examples of shock, as defined by Webster, is "a sudden or violent mental or emotional disturbance." Violent, emotional distress pretty much summed up my mind-set, but nausea, immobility, and tightening of my chest describe the physical reaction I had as I laid eyes on the woman they pointed to. I covered my mouth with my hand trying, trying to hold back a wave of queasiness.

Yes, this woman had on the same clothes as Mom did earlier, but that couldn't possibly be her. This individual was slumped over in her chair, head hung low, drool dripping from her mouth. I thought for a second I was looking at my grandmother. The person I'd left just a few hours earlier sat erect in the wheelchair, able to hold her head up, and never drooled. I ran to the wheelchair and kneeled in front of her, lifting her head up so that she could see me. I gently spoke her name: "Mom."

Her eyes were glassy as they locked onto mine, and she didn't utter a word. Her face looked somehow different, unresponsive, and expressionless. "What happened?" I asked out loud to the aides who were feeding other residents. "What happened to my mom? Something is wrong here." My emotions escalated alongside my voice as I looked around for someone else to help me. Refusing to let go of Mom's head, I shouted "Please, can someone help me?"

One of the aides left the resident they were feeding and came over to us. By this time, I was crying and my tone accusatory. "What happened to my mom?" I asked again, hating to make a scene in front of all the other residents but unable to stop myself.

Soon we were joined by the floor nurse and several others who appeared out of the woodwork. I repeated my questions, explaining that when I'd left her, she wasn't in this state. Something happened between the period I last saw her in the ambulance and finding her here. They looked confused, and the nurse stated they didn't know her before she arrived. "Your mom arrived in this condition," she explained. I looked around and my eyes fell on a couple of nearby residents slumped in wheelchairs, and I understood their explanation.

As my eyes returned to Mom, a visual played out in my mind. She was lying flat on a stretcher, taken out of her familiar environment, and placed inside a small foreign enclosure—the ambulance. Strangers surrounded her. Strapped in, she couldn't move her arms or legs. Her eyes darted around, coming to rest on a person sitting next to her. Who was he and where was Marianne? She opened her mouth, but nothing came out. What was happening? Confusion gave way to fear, and it shot through her like a tornado ripping through a small town, tearing down precious brain structures that were already severely compromised.

It was a scenario I hadn't considered. With all the planning and preparations, I had overlooked the impact of the transport. We deemed an ambulance the safest mode, and it was under a ten-minute drive, but to Mom it must have been the most terrifying ten minutes of her life. Guilt, brewing up like hot molten lava racing toward the top of a volcano, overflowed as I realized I'd abandoned my mom in her hour of need. I was the one responsible, not these individuals who were just trying to do their jobs. Why didn't I ask for help with the move, instead of once again thinking I could do it on my own?

Mom was evaluated by the head nurse and hospice the following day. It was later deemed she most likely suffered some form of a stroke while being transported. Arriving late afternoon, unaccompanied, and received by staff members who didn't have her history, Mom's condition wasn't questioned.

I spent the night on the floor by Mom's bed, mostly staring up at the ceiling and questioning my lack of sensitivity in planning. How had I not considered that the trip might push her over the edge? I would never intentionally hurt my mom, but I knew my lack of awareness contributed to her now weakened state. I was convinced my racing thoughts would never cease, and I would lie awake all night, but sleep finally found me and I awoke to a light knocking on the door. An aide arrived to help Mom get up and ready for the day. I noticed Mom was already stirring as I got up from the floor. She didn't speak, but she smiled as I said good morning. This was a good sign. Things were looking up a bit.

※ ※ ※

The new facility turned out to be a warm and caring sanctuary for Mom. The staff were compassionate and accommodating. The memory care unit was located on the lower walkout level in the back of the building, which made it easy to walk Mom around the path on nice days. It wasn't as swanky as the place she had just left behind, but it exuded more of a homey warmth—exactly what Mom needed during that time.

I met Mom in the mornings, and we'd spend the days in memory care listening to Christmas music, reading, saying the rosary, and taking walks. She frequently napped in her wheelchair. They had a friendly, loving dog in residence who made his way around the common area, laying his head on the lap of anyone in his path. He certainly captured hearts as he looked up with big, expressive eyes, always begging to be pet. Mom was an avid dog lover and would spot him moving toward her. He would rest his big loppy head in her lap, and she would try to move her hand toward him. She couldn't though because, since the move, her arms remained bent at the elbows and crossed over her chest. Her hands were clenched into fists, which brought back memories of my grandmother in that same position. Mom looked to be hugging herself, protecting the most vulnerable part of her body, her heart. I couldn't help but feel she was shielding herself from further onslaught.

Several times during her stay, Mom was treated to arm and hand massages as they tried to work those stiff limbs out. The therapist spoke tenderly while soft music played in the background; it usually relaxed her to the point of sleep. She was not able to hold her head up, so mealtimes were difficult as I held up her head with one hand and spoon fed her with the other. She wasn't eating much, only a few bites of soft foods, and we were thickening her liquids so that she wouldn't aspirate. Eventually, the only thing she would eat was the soft serve ice cream. I knew she didn't mind.

It was a heartbreaking period, but there was a surreal tranquility surrounding us amid the suffering. I sensed it without an awareness of what I was experiencing. I now know we were inching up on the diaphanous veil that separates our earthly existence from the next. Much like the gentle drizzle that covers everything in the proximity of a powerful waterfall, we were misted by serenity as we tottered on the edge of two worlds. We were metaphorically in liminal space.

Eleven days into the move, my niece (Mom's granddaughter), Becky, was getting married in Atlanta. On Thursday afternoon, the day before her wedding, Becky, my sister-in-law Margaret, and nephew Colin visited Mom. I could see by their pained expressions that they were shocked by Mom's appearance.

That evening, Steve and I settled Mom into bed for the night. I sat on the side of her bed as Steve sat in a nearby chair, working on his computer. Sitting quietly, I was watching Mom fall asleep when suddenly she opened her eyes and looked up at me. She spoke in a small, but discernable voice—a voice that hadn't uttered a single word since the move and couldn't string a complete sentence together for many months. Although she was looking at me, she was also looking beyond me as she said, "You are surrounded by beautiful people." I was stunned by her ability to speak but even more blown away by the passionate inflection in her voice. I covered my mouth with my hand, speechless, yet at the same time experiencing a consolation as if wrapped within a warm, cozy blanket.

I looked around, but the only other person in the room was Steve, and he was out of Mom's line of vision. Was she referring to my family who figuratively surrounded me? Yes, I was surrounded by beautiful people, but did she even remember them and their relationship to me? Did she remember me in as far as who I was in relationship to her?

Overhearing Mom, Steve got up and sat on the other side of the bed. Mom then began pointing to the wall behind us and in an excited voice exclaimed, "Look at all of those people." Steve and I looked behind us, but no one was there. Mom and Steve had a playful relationship, often trading jibes. He asked her in a teasing way to describe those people and she answered, "They are white."

Thunderstruck, Steve and I looked at each other then back at Mom. Both of us were present when our respective fathers passed away, but we'd never experienced anything like this. Not only was Mom lucid and speaking in sentences which hadn't happened in quite some time but she was seeing things—ghosts, it seemed—that we couldn't see. By this point in our journey, I didn't need any convincing that Mom existed beyond her failing brain but, witnessing her remarkable coherence and hearing her speak again, Mom was back! There was so much in that moment, and I wanted her to keep talking—looking at me like she knew me as her daughter and describing everything she saw that our eyes could not. "Please tell me more," I quietly pleaded. This was it, the apex of everything I sought from the beginning of Mom's journey and the validation that her sweet soul—there all along—was finally able to break through the massive wreckage in her brain. I envisioned her neural cells lighting up in jubilation as they reconnected with each other, wrapping up their earthly mission in one grand finale of a sublime yet worldly display that only our ears could grasp. And I wanted it to continue, but she fell back asleep. Steve and I left the building but couldn't leave behind what we had just experienced. We relived that wonder until the wee hours—analyzing and speculating—but mostly wishing she had said more about what she saw beyond these borders.

Friday morning arrived, and, while Mom and I were sitting in memory care, Juli came by to check on her. Still caught up in the phenomenon of the night before, my description of what had transpired gushed from my mouth before she could even utter a "good-morning!" Juli's eyes widened as her brows arched, and she went on to explain that she'd previously worked with hospice patients.

"These types of occurrences," she said, "often occur when patients are close to death. They report sightings, which some identify as loved ones, shortly before they pass." It was her belief that the presences they were seeing, and often having conversations with, were deceased family members and friends hovering near, preparing to accompany their loved one home. "I am shocked to hear this because your mom seems stable, I didn't think she was that close." This was a bittersweet revelation because I understood that the miraculous breakthrough I'd just enjoyed with Mom also meant she was near the very end of her journey.

I immediately called family members who had not come in town for the wedding and relayed Juli's message. Because these folks resided out of town, "How close?" was the question on everyone's mind. Unfortunately, that question was not easily or accurately answered, and, in Mom's case, she was still up and about in the wheelchair, eating, although not much, but certainly not in active dying.

In her present condition, according to Mom's hospice nurse, she could last for a month or possibly several. There was no formula, and everyone's path toward the end is different. It really is that hard to predict. Still, Juli's words about Mom's loved ones hovering close kept replaying in my mind. I think those words had the same effect on my brothers; those who could were making tentative plans to travel to Atlanta.

Saturday morning, the day after the wedding, I arrived midmorning to find Mom still sleeping in bed. I woke her slowly. She seemed exhausted and appeared much weaker than the night before. I alerted the staff and they tried to get her out of bed but were not able to get her to sit up. For the first time in all my years of memory, Mom did not get out of bed. She came from strong stock and not much kept her down. Because she now appeared to be rapidly declining, around the clock hospice was ordered and once again calls went out to my brothers. Mike, who had come in for the wedding on Friday, travelled back at first light Saturday morning and was nearing his home in Florida when he got the call.

Mom seemed to have taken a sharp downward turn, and, although hospice didn't think the end was imminent, I sensed it was. Over the course of the day other family members who had been in town for the wedding began filtering in. My oldest son, Ryan, was in the military and had been away for some time. When he walked in the room, Mom perked up and said, "Where have you been?" Amazingly, she was still speaking. My daughter-in-law, Jody, later told us that Mom was talking about beautiful people surrounding her and Ryan as they sat with her and that they too could not see. She remembers to this day the sensation of being held in an unexplainable yet extraordinary space.

Later that afternoon, as a few of us sat next to her bed and before the rest of my brothers arrived, Mom looked over at me and in a forceful voice emphatically asked, "Where are your brothers?" Mom was waiting for her family to arrive, and sure enough, as they filed in one by one over the course of the late evening and early morning hours, she woke up and acknowledged their presence. She had gained a mystifying clarity that is typical with terminal lucidity.

My family maintained a vigil during the overnight hours as she peacefully slept. The floor was littered with blankets, pillows, and sleeping bags that my husband brought from the house, but no one really slept—not even my brothers who had driven through the night. We all wanted to be present and assist Mom on this side of her journey, encouraging her and holding her hand as she prepared to leave that which is known and step into that which is not.

It is a humbling experience but also an extraordinary responsibility to be with a loved one as their time on this earth ticks down as heart-wrenching or bittersweet as those final days or hours may be. Watching her chest rise and fall, knowing that the beautiful air we share, the air that sustains all life on this side, will be hers for only a short time more. Remembering that she was there as we breathed our first breaths, we were grateful for the immense privilege to be with her as she took her last. The circle of life—beginnings and endings, hellos and goodbyes—was converging.

The long night gave way to a beautiful Sunday morning and Mom was still sleeping peacefully. Ryan and Jody ran into our pastor after Mass and let him know that Mom was dying. Father Nathan and Deacon Mark stopped by to administer Last Rites and to pray over Mom. Mom was a lifelong Catholic and this sacrament was very important to her; this final rite absolved her from any remaining sins, clearing the way for her soul to enter heaven. In the eyes of the Catholic Church, Mom was ready to meet her Maker.

We were told that hearing is the last of the senses to go and that the dying patient is very sensitive to loud noises. We spent the rest of Sunday quietly around Mom's bed as she peacefully slept, gently affirming her, and recalling happy and funny memories. We took turns leading the rosary and the Divine Mercy Chaplet as soft music played in the background.

The sun was beginning to form its long afternoon shadows, and, believing that Mom was still some ways off from active dying, Steve, my son Brady, and my brother Tim left to pick up dinner. I sat on one side of Mom, holding her hand, and my brother Kevin sat on the other, doing the same. The room was silent, and she was breathing peacefully.

Within a half hour of my family leaving however, Mom's breathing changed and started to become labored. Kevin and I looked over at each other, having been told by hospice that this change begins the final transition into active dying. Not knowing how long we had, we called the rest of the group and told them to hurry back. Her respiration then began to slow down and there were long pauses between breaths. Kevin ran to get the hospice nurse who came in and checked Mom. She informed us that the end was very near.

We affirmed Mom again, telling her it was OK to let go and that we loved her. We assured her we would be OK without her, wanting to give her the gift of peace as she departed. The rest of the family rushed in and formed a close circle around her bed. Everyone was touching some part of Mom's body, wanting that last physical connection to this matriarch who had led and loved us all so well. Then, through our tears, we pleaded with her to let go. And shortly after sunset on December 14, thirteen days after she arrived at Sun-Up, her beautiful, weathered old hands relaxed in ours, slid from our tight grip, and embraced the waiting hands of God.

※ ※ ※

Sleep well loved soul into the night;
The mission's complete, you're cleared for flight.
Your soul emerged here, so pure and sweet,
But as you journeyed, strife you did meet.
You accepted the work your Creator assigned;
The ebb and flow He thoughtfully designed.
It's part of the plan, your soul He did grow;
Until it perfected, then your body let go.
Your history's a treasure for loved ones to see;
Exam the artifacts, they're all meant to be.
Your life brings new meaning, as they journey along;
You're alive and well in the lyrics of their song.
Your flight plan's established, to the heavens you'll soar;
Pain free and peaceful, with God forevermore.
Sleep well loved soul into the night;
Your mission's complete, you're cleared for flight.

Written by me in the weeks following Mom's death.

Chapter Thirty-Five

Shortly after Sunset

14 December 2014

Of all the ways to lose a person, death is the kindest.
Ralph Waldo Emerson

Stillness blanketed the room as the moments hung in the gap between Mom's last breath and our ability to grasp the void. Thoughts vanished into nothingness; a numbness gave way to an open, lonely space. Something immeasurably big was gone.

Gradually, the exhaustion of Mom's final days, and the realization of her absence flooded my consciousness and emotions quickly commandeered the ship. If Mom had been hooked up to a heart monitor, the last spike of her EKG descending into a flat continuous line would have revealed the story behind the scenes; her heart abandoning its lifelong mission of delivering life-sustaining blood and oxygen throughout her body.

Because Mom was in hospice, no extraordinary means were employed during active dying other than to keep the patient comfortable, and in Mom's case that was liquid morphine drops placed inside her upper lip. We were told this small amount decreased respiratory distress by reducing the buildup of fluid in her lungs, easing what many call "gasping for breath." Mom calmly exhaled her last breath, our only indication of her soul slipping into the night, followed by the lack of a pulse.

I glanced around her last residence. Unpacked boxes by the window overflowing with prized possessions, window treatments with matching pillows strewn on the floor. Family pictures stacked in the corner still waiting to be hung; telltale signs of an abrupt move to a place where she never settled in. There were to-go cups and empty fast-food bags on the tables. Backpacks, pillows, and sleeping bags littered the floor, but Mom was the only one who slept.

This intimate gathering of family members communed as we recalled stories from the past, laughing and crying during one of life's most personal and bonding experiences—the passing of a loved one from this world. I looked at my husband, my brothers, my son. No words were spoken, but the physical and emotional fatigue from escorting Mom into the next life was unmistakably visible on their faces.

Death was indeed kind to Mom; she experienced a swift and peaceful passing. We instructed her to go toward those beautiful people she reported seeing only days earlier. Her last moments could be likened to a foot race where the end is in sight, but the steps to the finish are suspended in time. It seemed an eternity as we pleaded for Mom to take her last breath, but, when she did, her still warm body relaxed, and that familiar face softened as her spirited soul escaped.

In some ways dying is comparable to giving birth. It is laborious coming into this life and often equally so going out. Sometimes the struggle with dying is lengthy, beginning years before the final departure, especially with conditions like dementia and cancers. I have experienced the labor involved in giving birth and have witnessed the struggle that accompanies dying. I appreciate the toil for what it represents on both sides—the preparation for a new beginning—and Mom's entry into eternity was certainly that!

We were told the staff of the funeral home had arrived and were waiting on us to say our final goodbyes. With a life-ending disease like Alzheimer's, one slowly prepares for the end, but even when possibly ready, and knowing it's for the best, the final exhale is hard. I had let go of Mom in a million different ways as she became my aunt, cousin, or friend, but, in the end, she returned as my mom—and that's who I ultimately had to release.

My eyes rested on her sweet face, but if my vision could traverse the spiritual dimension, I imagined her casting one last loving glance on her family before being whisked away! The skies opened as she entered an expanse of majestic mountains topped with gleaming white snow. Weightless and soaring free, her spirit absorbed crystal-clear mountain lakes and lush green meadows filled with every color of wildflowers. Mom's idea of paradise!

In her final mission of mothering souls through this world, she confirmed our belief in the continuation of life beyond these borders. As Fr. Richard Rohr wrote about his mother in his *Continuum of Life* meditation,[46] Mom too built a bridge behind her as she spoke of those beautiful people only she could see. It was an assurance that she was not alone as she journeyed ahead and an invitation to bravely follow when it's our time to let go. The journey was not a sprint or marathon, but a relay, and I know that now I hold the baton.

Epilogue

The years teach us much which the days never knew.
Ralph Waldo Emerson

I have undertaken many journeys in my life. Travelling the path as a daughter and sister will be the longest, while wife, mother, and friend are a close second. Some of these trips are a flash in time although their impact may endure for a lifetime. Some are fun and easy, others challenging and painful. The latter are visitors with much to teach and will continue to return in some form until I've mastered their lessons. Occasionally I piggyback on the journeys of others as was the case with my mom and grandmother. They walked those grueling paths alone, but, ultimately and especially with Mom, I was the recipient of wisdom slowly unveiled in the rear-view mirror.

I began this journey asking if Mom existed beyond her brain damage. This was not a medical question although I found health care professionals willing to share what they had observed and ultimately came to believe about the existence of our beings beyond Alzheimer's. Like most other life-altering or life-ending diseases, Alzheimer's is a byproduct of our humanity; our physical organism gets sick and dies. But what lies beyond?

The feisty soul I came to know as Mom took up residence in a microscopic form after conception and continued after Alzheimer's. Mom thundered against the ruthlessness of the unseen assailant who stole her mother before it turned its greedy eyes on her. Despite a failing brain, she battled with every ounce of her being to remain relevant and enjoy life, fighting tirelessly for me to recognize her in that chaos.

While Alzheimer's nearly destroyed Mom during its initial encounter with my grandmother, it equally fortified her resolve to never submit to it. That doggedness didn't come from her body; it came from her soul. When God breathed life into that beautiful existence, he was exceptionally generous with determination as anyone who knew her will attest.

There are many definitions as well as types of faith, and my human language is severely limited in its ability to describe my innermost being much less comprehend the full scope of its eternal significance. But I innately know it's there, in that hiddenness, where in my most humble, vulnerable, and sometimes broken state I touch upon and draw from the vastness of God.

Initially, I sought to hold onto my mom as the person I had always known, the mother she had always been to me. Later, when it became apparent that she was not coming back to me in that form, I prayed to see her beyond her brain deterioration, beyond what was now missing—which was a big ask—as what I requested couldn't be seen with human eyes. I can't physically show a picture of a soul or whatever preferred word represents our innermost being. The closest for me comes down to the definition in Hebrews 11:1: "Now faith is the assurance of things hoped for, the conviction of things not seen."

Hoping did not get me what I asked for, not in the form I initially sought, and there was no guarantee I would see Mom in any form besides the demented one. But at some point during our journey, I realized that my conviction of a God I knew existed with every ounce of my being—without seeing—could also be true in reverse for a mom that I could see but no longer recognize. I had to wipe away old programming of how I perceived reality, which up until then was only with my five senses, and remain open to the mystery that lies beyond—the conviction of things not seen. And what was not seen until Mom's final days—but felt and sensed in awe—was that Mom was ever-present and that she had never left. That was my assurance of things hoped for.

Mom's dementia was the avenue I travelled that transformed my faith, but her determination was the instrument God used to nudge me along—her inexhaustible spirit that roared, "See me, see me, see me!" As Pierre Teilhard de Chardin so beautifully states, "We are not human beings having a spiritual experience, we are spiritual beings having a human experience."[47] And my very human experiences of frustration, pain, heartache, challenges, and doubts—over time—birthed in me the recognition of the spiritual; the hallowed ground I'd been walking with Mom all along.

Alzheimer's destroyed Mom's brain—her capacity to think, to reason, to recognize others, even to speak—but it could never erase who she was at the deepest level. I recognized her fiery nature, love of fashion, the choice of pink in her clothes and on her lips. I saw her outgoing spirit as she meandered a room, engaging everyone in her path. She was there on the dance floor as she gracefully moved to the beat of the music. I felt her love in tender touches and the huge smiles bestowed when I entered a room. She was spotted in her affection for dogs, even in her last days in memory care when she struggled to caress the sweet one in residence. She appeared during our walks on sunny days when she paused and took in flowers—she always loved flowers. I found Mom in her expressive eyes when she was happy, angry, or sad.

Letting go of the Mom I knew was a painful process that brought an incredible freedom when I finally released her. It allowed me to discover her all over again, and to appreciate qualities likely missed when we both were so busy living our lives. Being at peace with who she had become also freed me from trying to make order out of our disorder, allowing life to unfold as it should. When I embraced that mindset, I was transported to destinations on Mom's itinerary. We sometimes landed in stressful and heartbreaking places, but it felt so good to relinquish the wheel. Finally, letting go did not mean losing hope, as I continued to read and research possibilities for a cure, which, although too late for Mom, I pray is close for others.

In her terminal lucidity, Mom returned to those souls she transported into this world, assuring us of her permanence throughout the ages. It may have been our last physical sighting of that ceaseless existence and the final assignment of her earthly expedition, but the lessons unveil even to this day.

Shortly after Sunset

Accompanying Mom through Alzheimer's was a class I never wanted to take. During the more arduous sections I often sought the Cliffs Notes—to get through it as quickly as I could, and with the least amount of hardship as possible—but that shortcut always led to failure. I understood the *why* of Mom's suffering with dementia because I knew what was going on in her brain, but through much of this journey I didn't understand the *where*—where we were being led in the mystery of the pain and heartache. I couldn't ascertain that because I mistakenly thought I was on my own to figure it all out—but I was never alone in that darkness, nor was Mom. When I realized that and let go of any expectations or resolutions around this disease and my ability to control it, and when I quit asking for explanations of *why* we ended up in painful places, then I began to trust the *who*, and consequently was able to follow God to where I did not know to go. Only then was I able to detect the light—her beautiful and ceaseless soul—whenever it broke through. And there—in that brilliant manner of recognition—I could see Mom—and there she was—still dancing!

Dance on Mom!

Endnotes

Prologue

[1] Mitchell Colver, "Why Does Great Music Give You the Chills?" *Slate*, May 25, 2016, https://slate.com/technology/2016/05/getting-chills-when-listening-to-music-might-mean-youre-a-more-emotional-person.html.

[2] George Paxinos, "Why Psychology Lost Its Soul: Everything Comes from the Brain," *The Conversation*, September 22, 2016, https://theconversation.com/why-psychology-lost-its-soul- everything-comes-from-the-brain-54828.

Chapter One

[3] "The Power of Sankofa," *Berea College*, https://www.berea.edu/centers/carter-g-woodson- center-for-interracial-education/the-power-of-sankofa.

[4] Ana Lloret, Daniel Esteve, Maria-Angeles Lloret, Ana Cervera-Ferri, Begoña Lopez, Mariana Nepomuceno, and Paloma Monllor, "When Does Alzheimer's Really Start? The Role of Biomarkers," *International Journal of Molecular Sciences*, 20(22):5536 (2019), doi: 10.3390/ijms20225536.

[5] "The Later Stage of Dementia," *Alzheimer's Society*, last reviewed June 18, 2021, https://www.alzheimers.org.uk/about-dementia/symptoms-and-diagnosis/how-dementia-progresses/later-stages-dementia.

Chapter Two

[6] Emotions Can Affect Your Memory–Here's Why and How to Handle It. Medically reviewed by Matthew Boland, PhD–By Emily Swaim on July 10, 2022. https://www.healthline.com/health/mental-health/how-does-emotion-impact-memory#how-emotions-act-on-memory.

Chapter Three

[7] "Milestones," *Alzheimer's Association*, https://www.alz.org/alzheimers-dementia/research_progress/milestones#first.

Chapter Four

[8] "Wandering," *Alzheimer's Association*, https://www.alz.org/help-support/caregiving/stages-behaviors/wandering.

[9] Jonathan Graff-Radford, "Sundowning: Late-day Confusion," *Mayo Clinic*, https://www.mayoclinic.org/diseases-conditions/alzheimers-disease/expert-answers/sundowning/faq-20058511.

[10] Jonathan Graff-Radford, "Sundowning: Late-day Confusion," *Mayo Clinic*, https://www.mayoclinic.org/diseases-conditions/alzheimers-disease/expert-answers/sundowning/faq-20058511; William D. Todd, "Potential Pathways for Circadian Dysfunction and Sundowning-Related Behavioral Aggression in Alzheimer's Disease and Related Dementias," https://www.ncbi.nlm.nih.gov/pmc/articles/PMC7494756/.

[11] Denis Pare, Drew B. Headley, "The amygdala mediates the facilitating influence of emotions on memory through multiple interacting mechanisms," last reviewed May 24, 2023, https://www.ncbi.nlm.nih.gov/pmc/articles/PMC10034520/.

Chapter Five

[12] Amanda Wiggins and Jessica L. Bunin, "Confabulation," *StatPearls*, last reviewed August 28, 2023, https://www.ncbi.nlm.nih.gov/books/NBK536961/.

[13] Heidi Godman, "Above-Normal Blood Sugar Linked to Dementia," *Harvard Heath Blog*, August 7, 2013, https://www.health.harvard.edu/blog/above-normal-blood-sugar-linked-to-dementia-201308076596.

Chapter Six

[14] Hanns Hippius and Gabriele Neundörfer, "The Discovery of Alzheimer's Disease," *Dialogues in Clinical Neuroscience* 53.1 (2003), 101-08, https://www.ncbi.nlm.nih.gov/pmc/articles/PMC3181715/.

[15] "Milestones," *Alzheimer's Association*, https://www.alz.org/alzheimers-dementia/research_progress/milestones#first.

Chapter Eight

[16] Michael Nahm, Bruce Greyson, Emily Williams Kelly, and Erlendur Haraldsson " Terminal Lucidity: A Review and a Case Collection," *Archives of Gerontology and Geriatrics* 55.1 (2012), 138-142, https://doi.org/10.1016/j.archger.2011.06.031; Caitlin Geng, "What to Know About Terminal Lucidity and Dementia," *Medical News Today*, last reviewed August 30, 2022, https://www.medicalnewstoday.com/articles/terminal-lucidity-dementia.

[17] Ibid.

Chapter Ten

[18] Alvin Powell interviewing Rudolph Tanzi, "'New Clarity' against Alzheimer's," *Harvard Gazette*, May 5, 2015, https://news.harvard.edu/gazette/story/2015/05/new-clarity-against-alzheimers/.

[19] "Blood Test Can Predict Presence of Beta-Amyloid in the Brain, New Study Finds," *National Institute on Aging*, February 17, 2022, https://www.nia.nih.gov/news/blood-test-can-predict-presence-beta-amyloid-brain-new-study-finds.

[20] "What Happens to the Brain in Alzheimer's Disease," *National Institute on Aging*, last reviewed January 19, 2024. https://www.nia.nih.gov/health/alzheimers-causes-and-risk-factors/what-happens-brain-alzheimers-disease.

[21] Tim Tedeschi, "UC Study: Decreased Proteins, Not Amyloid Plaques, Tied to Alzheimer's Disease," *UC News*, October 4, 2022, https://www.uc.edu/news/articles/2022/09/decreased-proteins-not-amyloid-plaques-tied-to-alzheimers.html.

[22] Yasemin Saplakoglu, "What Causes Alzheimer's? Scientists Are Rethinking the Answer," *Quanta Magazine*, December 8, 2022, https://www.quantamagazine.org/what-causes-alzheimers-scientists-are-rethinking-the-answer-20221208/.

[23] Alzheimer's Study Explains How Tau Pathology Affects Brain Cells, July 29, 2021. Brian C. Kraemer, PhD, Pamela J. McMillan, PhD, C. Dirk Keene, MD, PhD, Caitlin Latimer, MD, PhD https://depts.washington.edu/mbwc/news/article/nuclear-speckles.

[24] Dick Benson interviewing Dale Bredesen, "Conversation with Dale Bredesen," *Integrative Medicine: A Clinician's Journal* 20.5 (2021): 44-47, https://www.ncbi.nlm.nih.gov/pmc/articles/PMC8594968/;

Craig Gustafson interviewing Dale Bredesn, "Dale E. Bredesen, MD: Reversing Cognitive Decline." *Integrative Medicine: A Clinician's Journal* 14.5 (2015): 26-29, https://www.ncbi.nlm.nih.gov/pmc/articles/PMC4712873/.

[25] "Foods that Fight Inflammation." *Harvard Health Publishing*, November 16, 2021 https://www.health.harvard.edu/staying-healthy/foods-that-fight-inflammation.

[26] "How Sleep Clears the Brain." *National Institute of Health*, October 28, 2013, https://www.nih.gov/news-events/nih-research-matters/how-sleep-clears-brain.

CHAPTER ELEVEN

[27] "Anosognosia," *Cleveland Clinic*, last reviewed April 21, 2022, https://my.clevelandclinic.org/health/diseases/22832-anosognosia.

[28] "What Is Mild Cognitive Impairment?," *National Institute on Aging*, last reviewed April 12, 2021, https://www.nia.nih.gov/health/what-mild-cognitive-impairment.

CHAPTER THIRTEEN

[29] Rebecca M Bollinger, Audrey Keleman, Regina Thompson, Elizabeth Westerhaus, Anne M Fagan, Tammie LS Benzinger, Suzanne E Schindler, Chengjie Xiong, David Balota, John C Morris, Beau M Ances, and Susan L Stark, "Falls: A Marker of Preclinical Alzheimer Disease: A Cohort Study Protocol," *BMJ Open* 11.9 (2021), doi: 10.1136/bmjopen-2021-050820.

[30] "State Regulations on Dementia and Driving," https://adsd.nv.gov/uploadedFiles/adsdnvgov/content/Boards/TaskForceAlzheimers/State%20Regulations%20Dementia%20and%20Driving.pdf;

JAMA Network Open, published online January 5, 2024, NIH, National Library of Medicine, Reporting Requirements, Confidentiality, and Legal Immunity for Physicians Who Report Medically Impaired Drivers, Elaine

M. Tran, MD., and Jeffrey E. Lee, MD. https://www.ncbi.nlm.nih.gov/pmc/articles/PMC10770772/#:~:text=Six%20states%20had%20mandatory%20reporting,impaired%20drivers%20confidential%20without%20exception.

Chapter Fourteen

[31] Jonathan Graff-Radford, "Ministroke vs. Regular Stroke: What's The Difference?" *Mayo Clinic*, April 14, 2023, https://www.mayoclinic.org/diseases-conditions/transient-ischemic-attack/expert-answers/mini-stroke/faq-20058390.

[32] "GP Records Indicate Long Term Effects on Patients of 'Mini-Strokes,'" *University of Birmingham*, July 20, 2016, https://www.birmingham.ac.uk/news-archive/2016/gp-records-indicate-long-term-effects-on-patients-of-mini-strokes-1.

Chapter Fifteen

[33] "Sleep Deprivation Increases Alzheimer's Protein," *National Institutes of Health*, April 24, 2018, https://www.nih.gov/news-events/nih-research-matters/sleep-deprivation-increases-alzheimers-protein.

[34] Tianna Hicklin, "Gene Identified in People Who Need Little Sleep," *National Institutes of Health*, September 17, 2019, https://www.nih.gov/news-events/nih-research-matters/gene-identified-people-who-need-little-sleep.

[35] "Luckiest Man," *National Baseball Hall of Fame*, https://baseballhall.org/discover-more/stories/baseball-history/lou-gehrig-luckiest-man.

Chapter Sixteen

[36] Annie Lennon, "Reading, Writing, and Playing Games Delay Alzheimer's by 5 Years," *Medical News Today*, July 19, 2021, https://www.medicalnewstoday.com/articles/reading-writing-and-playing-games-delay-alzheimers-by-5-years#Making-the-brain-more-resilient.

[37] "The 7 Stages of Alzheimer's Disease," *Penn Medicine Neuroscience Blog*, December 31, 2020, https://www.pennmedicine.org/updates/blogs/neuroscience-blog/2019/november/stages-of-alzheimers.

Chapter Eighteen

[38] "What Does an Older Adult Law Attorney Do?," *FindLaw*, last reviewed August 2, 2023, https://www.findlaw.com/elder/what-is-elder-law/what-does-an-elder-law-attorney-do-.html.

[39] Henry Vaughn, "The Revival," https://www.luminarium.org/sevenlit/vaughan/revival.htm.

Chapter Nineteen

[40] Center for Action and Contemplation, Love and Suffering, August 14, 2022, Father Richard Rohr, https://cac.org/daily-meditations/love-and-suffering-2022-08-14/.

[41] Ibid.

Chapter Twenty-Two

[42] Andrea Matthews, "What Does It Mean to Let Go?," *Psychology Today*, March 12, 2016, https://www.psychologytoday.com/us/blog/traversing-the-inner-terrain/201603/what-does-it-mean-let-go.

Chapter Twenty-Eight

[43] "Dementia: Addressing the Stigma of America's Most Feared Diagnosis," *Milken Institute*, June 22, 2021, https://milkeninstitute.org/video/dementia-addressing-stigma.

https://milkeninstitute.org/video/dementia-addressing-stigma

Chapter Thirty

[44] Joe Nuxhall, Cincy, June, 2019, https://www.cincymagazine.com/rounding-third-and-heading-for-home/#.

[45] Daniel Miller, "What is Anticipatory Grief?" *Psychology Today*, March 1, 2022, https://www.psychologytoday.com/us/blog/end-life-matters/202203/what-is-anticipatory-grief.

Chapter Thirty-Five

[46] Center for Action and Contemplation, Fr Richard Rohr, The Continuum of Life, October 30, 2022, https://cac.org/daily-meditations/the-continuum-of-life-2022-10-30/.

Epilogue

[47] Pierre Teilhard de Chardin, *OneJourney*, https://onejourney.net/pierre-teilhard-de-chardin-we-are-not-human-beings-having-a-spiritual-experience.

Milton Keynes UK
Ingram Content Group UK Ltd.
UKHW012131110624
443988UK00001B/87